PEOPLE ARE TALKING ABOUT *THE NEW LEAN FOR LIFE*!

"My weight was an issue my entire life. I was convinced I would live—and die—as a fat person. But when a friend lost 65 pounds on the Lean for Life program, I got inspired. The last year has been truly life-changing. I've lost 90 pounds. I've gotten my life back!"–**KATE, 39**

"I was sick and tired of feeling sick and tired. I committed to becoming Lean for Life—and I did. I lost 28 pounds in 10 weeks, and I've kept it off for three years!"–**RACHELE, 27**

"I'm a man of few words, so when people notice my 66-pound weight loss and ask me how I did it, I have a five-second answer that says everything. I tell them, 'I did the Lean for Life program. It's fast. It's easy. And it works.'"–**MICHAEL, 43**

"Before I did the Lean for Life program, I was on diabetes, cholesterol and blood pressure medication. Not anymore!"–**JESSE, 35**

"When I told my best friend I was doing the Lean for Life program, she said I looked just fine the way I was. But I knew how much healthier I looked and felt when I weighed less. To some people, 15 pounds is nothing. To me, it was everything!"–**BRIONNA, 19**

"After losing 42 pounds, it never occurred to me that I'd regain it! But life got busy, I got distracted and I gradually began reverting to old habits. Realizing I'd regained 20 pounds really annoyed me, but it didn't discourage me. I knew the Lean for Life program had worked for me once. There was no reason it wouldn't work for me again. And guess what? It did!"–**DOROTHY, 57**

"I grew up in a family in which everyone overate—and everyone is overweight. Once I made the connection that how I eat directly impacts how I look and feel, I decided to live differently. I committed to becoming Lean for Life, and I lost 54 pounds. I've maintained a healthy weight for nearly four years. Change isn't always easy, but it's easier than you think—and it's a lot easier than being fat!"–**AUSTIN, 26**

"There's a lot to love about the Lean for Life program, but what I valued most was the consistency and structure that it provided. The day-by-day approach helped me keep on track and eliminated the guesswork."–**JACKSON, 28**

"I lost 33 pounds, but what I've gained matters to me even more. I have so much more confidence and energy. Life is a lot more fun when you feel healthy!"–**SARAH, 41**

BOOKS BY CYNTHIA STAMPER GRAFF

LEAN FOR LIFE PHASE TWO: LIFETIME SOLUTIONS (Griffin Publishing Group, 2001)

LEAN FOR LIFE PHASE ONE: WEIGHT LOSS (Griffin Publishing Group, 2001)

LEAN FOR LIFE (Griffin Publishing Group, 1997)

BODYPRIDE (Griffin Publishing Group, 1997)

BOOKS BY RÉGINALD ALLOUCHE, M.D.

LE PLAISIR DU SUCRE AU RISQUE DU PRÉ-DIABÈTE [FROM SUGAR ADDICTION TO PREDIABETES RISK] (Editions Odile Jacob, 2013)

MINCIR À SATIÉTÉ [THINNESS THROUGH SATIETY] (Flammarion 2009)

LA RÉVOLUTION MINCEUR [THE THINNESS REVOLUTION] (Michel Lafon, 2003)

THE NEW LEAN FOR LIFE

**CYNTHIA STAMPER GRAFF
& RÉGINALD ALLOUCHE, M.D.**

Outsmart Your Body to Shrink Fat Cells and Lose Weight for Good

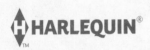

THE NEW LEAN FOR LIFE

ISBN-13: 978-0-373-89303-4
© 2014 by Cynthia Stamper Graff

Lean for Life is a registered trademark of Lindora LLC.
Lindora is a registered trademark of Lindora LLC.
BioMod is a registered trademark of Lindora LLC.
Stay-Weight is a registered trademark of Lindora LLC.
Capsio-Lin is a registered trademark of Lindora LLC.
Mitochondriac is a registered trademark of Lindora LLC.
Mr. Mito is a registered trademark of Lindora LLC.
KOT is a registered trademark of Ceprodi SA.

The health advice presented in this book is intended only as an informative resource guide to help you make informed decisions; it is not meant to replace the advice of a physician or to serve as a guide to self-treatment. Always seek competent medical help for any health condition or if there is any question about the appropriateness of a procedure or health recommendation.

Library of Congress Cataloging-in-Publication Data
Graff, Cynthia Stamper, 1953-
  The new lean for life : outsmart your body to shrink fat cells and lose weight for good / Cynthia Stamper Graff and Réginald Allouche, M.D.
      pages cm
  Includes bibliographical references and index.
  ISBN 978-0-373-89303-4 (alk. paper)
1. Reducing diets. 2. Weight loss—Psychological aspects. 3. Neuropsychology. I. Allouche, Réginald, 1956- II. Title.
  RM222.2.G682 2014
  613.2'5--dc23
                              2013027703

www.Harlequin.com

Printed in U.S.A.

*To our families and patients, and to Dr. Marshall Stamper
and the other pioneers in the field of obesity medicine
who had the strength of their convictions.
We'll carry on in their tradition.*

—Cynthia Stamper Graff and Réginald Allouche, M.D.

CONTENTS

INTRODUCTION

WHY *THE NEW LEAN FOR LIFE* WILL WORK FOR YOU, AND HOW TO USE THIS BOOK

How many times have you lost some weight while on a diet only to gain it all back later after you stopped the diet? Once? Twice? More times than you can count? You're not alone. Nearly half of all dieters quit within the first month. This dire statistic from a 2012 study reinforces the fact that *starting* a diet program is easy; *staying with it* is the hard part. Yet the only way a diet program is going to work for you is if you actually stick with it. Now what if a diet could anticipate what you are thinking as you progress from day to day? What if a program could actually *address* your feelings, frustrations and questions *as* you feel them, and also provide success strategies at the very moment you need them most so you can stay on your program and reach your goal weight?

After more than *15 million* visits with patients at the Lindora weight-loss clinics in Southern California, the Lean for Life program is able to do just that—using what we've learned from more than 750,000 people who have lost a combined 15 million pounds on our program in the past 40-plus years. We guide our patients on a day-by-day basis through four weeks of Rapid Weight Loss, easing them through the tough days and using the easier days to give them additional insights on what they need to know to succeed on the program to get lean and stay lean.

In just four weeks, our patients enjoy more than rapid weight loss; they get a blueprint to a leaner body, reduced stress levels, more balanced blood sugar levels and a new way of thinking—all in a simple, accessible program. An internal data analysis of Lean for Life patients found that 79 percent kept weight off and 43 percent maintained medically significant weight loss for up to 15 years after completing their program. Compare this to the widely quoted statistic that 95 percent of dieters typically regain the weight they worked so hard to lose on conventional diets. On this program, people really do get Lean for Life.

MORE THAN 750,000 SUCCESS STORIES... AND COUNTING!

You could say that I (Cynthia) grew up in the "waist-management" business. My father, weight-loss pioneer Marshall Stamper, M.D., opened his first Lindora weight-loss clinic in 1971. Motivated by the loss of his mother, who had died of obesity-related complications, Dr. Stamper created a comprehensive, results-oriented program that helped people lose weight rapidly and safely. At the foundation of the program were Dr. Stamper's Six Essentials, which taught people how to change their behavior and change their physiology, making it easier to maintain their new, healthier weight. Throughout this book, you'll discover more about the Six Essentials—which remain a cornerstone of the program—and how they can help you reach your weight-loss goals.

Decades ago, Dr. Stamper was convinced that if people lost weight and learned healthier thinking habits, they could reverse or prevent certain ailments and health conditions. At the time, people called it "woo-woo science." Today, it's common knowledge that being overweight is a factor in type 2 diabetes, heart disease, cancer and more. Dr. Stamper and his program were light years ahead of their time.

Back when I was a teenager, I was Dr. Stamper's guinea pig. In order to help me lose a few pounds, he put me on his revolutionary Rapid Weight Loss plan. It went far beyond ordinary meal plans and included a blueprint to "leanify" not just my body, but also my stress levels, my way of thinking and my daily habits. It helped me get lean and stay lean—not just for a few weeks or a couple of months as with most diets, but Lean for Life.

Over the past 40-plus years, this same program helped people ranging from Hollywood stars wanting to drop those last 5 pounds to others struggling to lose more than 500 pounds. We've helped people not only whittle their waistline but also get off their blood pressure, cholesterol, type 2 diabetes and pain medications. We've helped lifetime yo-yo dieters get off the weight-loss roller coaster and maintain their new lean weight for years. We've seen people transform their bodies and their lives. You'll meet many of these "Lean for Lifers" within the pages of this book, including:

- **Traci,** who lost more than 300 pounds and has kept it off for more than 10 years.

- **Kimberly,** who shrank from a size 18 to a sleek size 6.

- **Laura,** who dropped 36 pounds in 10 weeks and no longer has to take her cholesterol, blood pressure or type 2 diabetes medicines.

- **Javier,** who went from a 52-inch waist to a 34-inch waist.

So far, we have more than 750,000 success stories, and there's no stopping! Each year, 35,000 real-life, everyday people like Traci, Kimberly, Laura and Javier visit our 40-plus clinics located throughout Southern California for in-person appointments with our staff of healthcare professionals, which includes M.D.s and registered nurses. Since I joined forces with Dr. Stamper (affectionately known as "Daddy") in 1988, I've been trying to make it easier than ever for people everywhere—not just those who live close enough to visit our clinics—to lose weight with our program. As a result, people can now log on to our personalized, interactive web-based program for daily support anywhere, anytime. People everywhere can also track the calories and nutrient content of our nutritional products on top-selling diet apps like Lose It! Thousands of people have gotten lean thanks to our books and products, which are sold in pharmacies and other stores nationwide. And millions of people have access to our program through their membership with some of the nation's largest health insurance providers.

Finding new ways and new strategies to help as many people as possible become Lean for Life has been my number-one goal. That's why, in the mid-1990s, I distilled the basics of the Lean for Life program used in Lindora Clinics in my first book, *Lean for Life*. I wanted the book to be not only a daily support tool for our patients as they progressed through the program, but also a way to make the program available to the tens of thousands of people who couldn't visit our clinics in person and who wanted to lose weight at home...*but didn't want to do it on their own*. It worked, and more than a decade after its publication, that book was still ranked as one of the top-selling books on Amazon.com.

Since the original book was published, however, a growing body of weight-loss science has emerged. This exciting new research provides insights into ways to enhance the Lean for Life program and proves why this program is so effective, validating the foundation of the program that has already helped so many people reach their weight goals. More than a decade of new science, new breakthroughs, new strategies and new techniques convinced me it was time to refine the program and update the book.

That's where a box of cookies came into play.

HOW A BOX OF COOKIES INSPIRED
THE NEW LEAN FOR LIFE

In 2012, one of our Lean for Life patients returned from a vacation in Paris with a gift for me—a box of gourmet dark chocolate European tea biscuits. She told me they were incredibly delicious, and she couldn't wait to share them with me. I immediately buzzed our operations team and asked them to join me in the conference room. When they arrived, we broke open the box, peeled away the wrappers and started munching—assessing the flavors, the crunchiness of the delicate biscuits and the richness of the chocolate.

There we were, a team of weight-loss professionals, nibbling on a box of cookies at 10:30 in the morning. Any passerby would have thought we were a bunch of frauds. You may be wondering, why on earth would someone who has finally reached her ideal lean weight after failing on so many other diets bring me—the CEO of one of the nation's largest medically supervised weight-loss system—a box of cookies? And why would I encourage my staff to indulge in a mid-morning cookie-fest? It's not as crazy as it seems.

This was no ordinary box of cookies.

They were Europe's number-one brand of gourmet *diet* foods, and not only were they just as delicious as promised, but they were also formulated based on groundbreaking findings from the world of brain and satiety science, incorporating special nutrients known to enhance satiety and reduce hunger without sacrificing taste. Basically, they were engineered to accelerate weight loss while allowing you to eat the foods you've come to love. To say that I was intrigued is an understatement. After all, my mission is to find ways to make it easier for you to become Lean for Life.

A SMARTER PLAN TO OUTSMART YOUR BIOLOGY

With a little investigating, I soon learned who was behind those delicious European diet cookies. Réginald Allouche, M.D., is a diabetes and weight-loss specialist, one of the world's foremost nutrition experts and the founder of KOT, the top brand of gourmet diet foods in Europe. The KOT products—including crêpes, pizza, pancakes, cookies and even ice cream—are sold in 2,200 pharmacies throughout Europe and are used by more than 700,000 dieters there.

I was thrilled when Dr. Allouche accepted my invitation to come to our Southern California headquarters to meet with me and Dr. Stamper, who remains my most trusted advisor. Charming and effervescent, Dr. Allouche entertained us as he detailed his groundbreaking scientific research. He gave us a fascinating explanation of the inner workings of the brain, body and gut and how they gang up in overweight people to make it almost impossible to lose weight. Then he shared how he has spent his career trying to reverse that and get the brain, body and gut to help you lose weight. I'll let Dr. Allouche take it from here.

The Inside Story from Dr. Allouche

After more than 25 years as a practicing diabetes physician, I came to realize that type 2 diabetes isn't simply a blood sugar problem but also what I call a "brain decision." My fascination with the brain's role in type 2 diabetes sparked further research into how the brain is involved in satiety and weight gain, specifically, the connection between deprivation dieting and diet failure.

I observed that some of my overweight type 2 diabetic patients were unable to stick to the healthy diet I prescribed, even when it presented a risk to their lives not to do so. Amazingly, they reported that they would rather risk the devastating consequences of uncontrolled type 2 diabetes—blindness, painful nerve damage and even amputations—than give up their fat-laden croissants and sweet crêpes. One patient in particular proved especially challenging.

This patient, to whom we will refer as *Monsieur X*, was an overweight type 2 diabetic CEO of a major French corporation. I had been treating him for months, yet his weight and blood sugar levels remained high. Monsieur X complained that he had nothing to eat on the prescribed program, so I said, "Let's go to the grocery store, NOW!" As we went up and down the aisles of the supermarket I pointed out all the lean meats, fish, eggs, vegetables, fruits and whole grains that I had recommended. Monsieur X took one look at me and said, "You expect me to eat nothing but *that* for the rest of my life? If there's no pleasure in eating, then I'll never be able to stick to your plan, so why bother trying?"

That led to an epiphany. What if I could help people to eat the foods they love without ruining their healthy eating plan? Armed with postgraduate degrees in biological and medical engineering and a strong background in nutrition, I went to work.

I pored through the latest medical findings and zeroed in on a certain type of peptides—molecules found in proteins—that had proven to increase satiety and quell hunger for hours. Years of testing and tasting resulted in—*voilà*—a proprietary blend of milk-extracted peptides combined with soluble fibers to create high-protein, low-glycemic foods and snacks that provided the pleasure my patients were looking for while dramatically reducing hunger, protecting lean muscle mass and promoting weight loss. Clinical studies have shown that consuming the products while following a weight-loss program like Lean for Life shrinks fat cells twice as much as conventional diets.

As I like to say, "To win the battle of obesity and type 2 diabetes, I had to use the weapons of pleasure."

- -

After hearing Dr. Allouche talk about how he worked with his patients, Dr. Stamper felt an instant rapport with the French weight-loss innovator. The two of them shared a similar approach to caring for patients. Rather than viewing their patients as statistics or "the gall bladder in room 4," they viewed each patient as an individual, whose brain, body, environment, emotions and thought patterns contributed to their weight problems. And they both understood that in order to help patients lose the weight, they had to treat all of those factors.

The meeting was so successful that I eventually collaborated with Dr. Allouche in 2012 to incorporate his scientific findings about the brain, body and gut—as well as a touch of the French joie de vivre—into the Lean for Life program. The two of us spent months infusing the program with the latest science-based strategies to enhance its effectiveness and make it easier—and more *délicieux*—than ever to follow. And together, we rewrote the book that had already helped so many people achieve their weight-loss goals. The end result? *The New Lean for Life!*

WHAT'S NEW IN *THE NEW LEAN FOR LIFE?*

In this book, we've streamlined the Lean for Life program, incorporating Dr. Allouche's own groundbreaking research, as well as that of others. Did you know that—for your brain—weight loss and satiety go hand in hand? In *The New Lean for Life* you'll become an expert in satiety science and understand why deprivation dieting is doomed to fail, and why allowing you to eat the lip-smacking foods you would end up consuming anyway is essential for long-term weight loss. Our new program includes up-to-the-minute findings from the world of science that show how your brain, body and gut make you a slave to the habits that can supersize you. Then we give you a plan to trick your brain, body and gut into helping you change your habits and get lean instead.

You'll get to know how your brain and body can actually "forget" how to eliminate the contents of your fat cells, which causes you to keep stockpiling more and more excess fat, and discover our plan to help your brain and body remember how to release the fat from your fat cells. And there's so much more.

Here's what *The New Lean for Life* can do for you:

- Help you shrink the size of your fat cells—*twice as much as conventional diets!*
- Show you how to lose up to 20 pounds in 28 days.
- Allow you to enjoy more "forbidden" foods like cookies and pancakes and still lose weight.
- Reprogram your appetite so you won't feel hungry while losing weight.
- Rewire your brain so you can change the mindless everyday habits that are holding you back from reaching your weight goals.
- Heal your gut to calm cravings and improve satiety.

- Show you how to use "thought control" to fight the negative thoughts that sabotage your success.
- Curb cravings with our "Emergency Cravings Toolkit."
- Rev up metabolism with our "90-Second Fat-Burning Booster" exercise plan.
- Begin reversing fat-promoting health conditions, such as insulin resistance and chronic inflammation—*in just 2 weeks!*

Of course, as with the original program, we'll continue to hold your hand through the process and help you manage daily obstacles so you can be successful—not just for a month but for life!

Note: This is a powerful program. A ketogenic diet like Lean for Life is not recommended for type 1 insulin-dependent diabetics, pregnant or nursing mothers, or people with serious liver or kidney disease. Before starting this or any diet, it is recommended to seek advice from your personal healthcare provider. We encourage you to take the "A Message to Your Doctor" letter on page 286 with you to your healthcare provider.

HOW TO USE THIS BOOK

The New Lean for Life isn't a book you *read*; it is a book you *do*. It is a 28-day prescription to shrink your fat cells and shrink your body. It is intended to be a constant companion. Everything about the way this book is organized and presented is based on what we have found to be most helpful to our patients in their journey to rapid, lasting weight loss.

For example, in our experience, new dieters often feel overwhelmed by the "commitment" of reading several chapters of science before getting to the action plan that will help them begin losing weight. We've observed that our clinic patients don't want all that scientific information all at once about *why* they're overweight. They want to get started right away with *what to do* to get lean. That's why this book takes a completely different approach from what you may be used to. We call it the "drip method," and it simply means that we'll dole out new ideas and information about the overall program and the science behind it in small, bite-sized chunks that are easily digestible. Think of it as brain food! Chapters 4 through 7 are broken down into "daily doses" of this brain food.

Way more fun than Biology 101, chapter 1 features Dr. Allouche's look at how your brain, body and gut can conspire to transform what you eat into a "spare tire" or "muffin top." Forget about classroom science—Dr. Allouche will be providing you with "weird science," the kind you can actually put to use in the real world to help make you Lean for Life. Throughout the book, you'll find the latest science revealed in "The Inside Story from Dr. Allouche," where he explores what you can do to get your brain, body and gut working for you instead of against you.

The "start now" advice comes immediately after that in chapter 2, where we'll provide an overview of the plan and specifics on what you'll be eating and doing to shrink your fat cells and "leanify" your body. Chapter 3 details our three-day "Prep" that primes your brain, body and gut for optimal results. In chapters 4 through 7, which focus on the four weeks of Rapid Weight Loss, we'll guide you day by day, offering simple success strategies to help you cope with the many stumbling blocks you may encounter along the way. Chapter 8 details a critical two-week transition period that resets your metabolism so you can eat more *without gaining weight*. And chapter 9 gives you all the tools you need to stay Lean for Life.

For links to additional helpful tools on our website, look for the QR code, as seen in the "QR code" figure, throughout the book. To gain access to the information, you just need to open the QR Reader app on your Look for the QR code to access additional information on our website. mobile phone and hold your phone over the code. If you don't already have a QR Reader, you can download the app for free.

The New Lean for Life gives you so many new tools to help you get—and stay—lean that even if you're already a Lean for Life patient or have followed the original program at some point in the past, you'll benefit from the science-based solutions in this book. And if you're one of the millions of people who have started diet after diet but have had trouble sticking with it or have lost weight only to regain it, the simple strategies in this book will help you stay on the program so you can become Lean for Life.

So come along. Let's get started. I can't wait to share all of our secrets with you!

YOUR INSIDE STORY:

HOW YOUR BRAIN, BODY AND GUT CAN CONSPIRE TO TRANSFORM A SLICE OF PIZZA INTO A SPARE TIRE

When people first come to our clinics, it's often after they've already tried—and failed—to slim down on their own or with fad diets. Frustrated by their lack of success, they almost always ask us why it's so hard for them to lose weight and keep it off. "Is it my genetics? Is it because I can't control my cravings? Is it because I eat too many carbs? Is it because I eat when I'm stressed? Is it because there's a bakery next door to my office?" Unfortunately, there's no one single answer. In fact, the answer is usually more along the lines of: "all of the above…and more." After helping more than 750,000 people shed excess fat, we know that there are numerous psychological, behavioral, environmental and physiological processes at work. And we've found that, in terms of biology, your brain, body and gut can conspire to make you pile on pounds and make it difficult for you to lose weight.

To illustrate just how your brain, body and gut can collude to keep you fat, let's look at a slice of pizza. You like pizza, don't you? Most people love a good slice of pizza. But have you ever wondered what really happens to that slice after you bite into it? You know that it tends to end up on your hips, thighs and belly, but how? To demystify the process, Dr. Allouche is going to give you an inside look at what happens when you eat a slice of gooey, delicious pizza and follow that tasty morsel as it takes a fantastic voyage through your body. Along the way, you'll discover how your brain, body and gut can gang up to make it harder for you to lose weight, and more important, you'll get a glimpse of how the Lean for Life program will help you get them working for you again.

The Inside Story from Dr. Allouche

THE AMAZING JOURNEY OF A SLICE OF PIZZA

JUST FOR THE SMELL OF IT—AWAKENING YOUR BRAIN

The digestive process (see "The Digestive Tract") begins before you ever take a bite. Just seeing the melted cheese, inhaling the tantalizing aroma of the pepperoni topping and touching the crispiness of the crust alerts your brain that you are about to indulge in something really good: *Get ready brain, here it comes!* Within milliseconds, your brain fires off signals that trigger a number of chemical events in anticipation of that first delicious bite, causing your mouth to water, and your stomach to release small amounts of gastric acids.

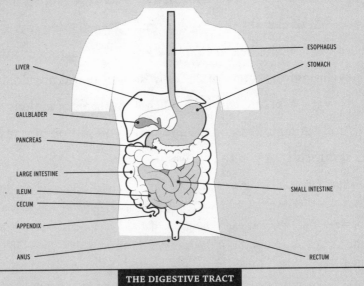

THE DIGESTIVE TRACT

In the human digestive tract, the brain, body and gut communicate with each other.

CHEWING THE FAT...AND PROTEIN AND CARBS

The second you slide that piece of pizza into your mouth, your incisors, canines and molars go to work. With the ability to produce 120 pounds of bite pressure, your teeth mash up that first bite so you can swallow it. Chewing your pizza also spreads it throughout your mouth, where your 5,000 or so taste buds pick up on a variety of flavors, including the saltiness of the pepperoni and the hint of sweetness from the sugar used in the tomato sauce (yes, there's sugar in most tomato sauces!). This prompts your salivary glands to pump out more saliva, which comingles with the food and coats it so it will slide down your esophagus more easily.

All that gnashing also triggers the release of digestive enzymes within the saliva, including one called *amylase*, which allows your body to assimilate carbohydrates, such as those in the crispy, golden pizza crust. Another enzyme called *lipase* immediately goes to work to break down the fats in the bubbling cheese and sliced pepperoni on your pizza.

One of the most important things chewing does is send signals to receptors in your brain and gut indicating that you're eating. This is critical because when your brain gets the message that you're eating, it starts putting the brakes on the hunger hormones that increase your appetite. And when your gut gets that *I'm not hungry* message, it prepares to produce the hormones that tell you *I'm full*. The longer you chew, the sooner your brain and gut get those messages, and the faster *you* get the message to say no to another slice of pizza.

But what happens for those of us who can't seem to stop at one helping?

WHEN THINGS GO WRONG

Some of us gulp down our food rather than chewing it thoroughly. Without a proper amount of chewing, your brain doesn't have a chance to get the message to halt production of your hunger hormones and your gut doesn't have the time it requires to produce enough of the hormones that indicate fullness. Because of this, you keep gulping down more food, and even though you're consuming larger quantities, you still feel hungry.

Another problem arises from eating foods that create a veritable flavor explosion in the mouth. Although some variety in your diet is required for optimal health, too much variety can lead to overeating. Your mouth relies on sensory stimuli, including aromas, textures and flavors, to send satiety signals to the brain. The human mouth loves all of these, and the more variety of them available, the more it wants to get its fill of each of them. If a variety of flavors, textures and aromas are jam-packed into one single food source—say, the crunchy crust, melted cheese, spicy tomato sauce and piquant pepperoni on your pizza—your mouth demands more of it to savor it all.

WHEN YOU'RE LEAN FOR LIFE

Throughout this book, you'll discover how to make simple changes in what you eat and the way you eat that put your hunger hormones on hold for hours, fire up production of the hormones that keep you feeling full and increase the satiety signals heading from your mouth to your brain. Now back to that slice of pizza.

YOUR ESOPHAGUS: DOWN SHE GOES!

When you're ready to swallow, your tongue pushes the mouthful of mashed-up contents in your mouth, called a *bolus*, toward the back of your throat and, *gulp!* As it enters your esophagus, a layer of smooth muscle within begins a series of involuntary undulating contractions, known as *peristalses*, that force the food downward. In only a matter of seconds, the food traverses the 10 inches of your esophagus to arrive at your stomach, which opens up to allow the pizza inside.

YOUR STOMACH: THE WORLD'S BEST BLENDER

Your stomach acts like a high-powered blender, breaking down the small bits of pizza into tinier and tinier pieces. To aid in this process, your stomach produces gastric juices, including hydrochloric acid, which is so corrosive that over time it could pickle steel. These juices not only pulverize the food particles but also kill the millions of potentially harmful bacteria that you consume with every bite.

Inside your stomach, an enzyme called *pepsin* begins the laborious process of breaking down those yummy pepperoni slices into tinier bits of protein called *peptides*. This process is known as *hydrolysis*, and protein that has been broken down into amino acids is referred to as *hydrolyzed protein*.

Just like when you put your blender on the "pulse" mode, your stomach muscles (which have absolutely nothing to do with the abdominal muscles you try to exercise at the gym) contract about every 20 seconds to churn up its contents. The blending, pulsing and contracting continues for about two to four hours. Sensors in your stomach relay information to your brain about the amount of pressure within based on the quantity of food in the mixer—the more food, the more pressure. When the pressure gets too high, your brain provokes spasms to push the food toward the exit.

Some parts of your pizza are easier to break down than others. The carbohydrate crust digests the fastest, followed by the fats and then the protein in the cheese and pepperoni.

After being puréed, the contents of your stomach resemble a liquefied blob, similar to what that piece of pizza would look like if you actually had tossed it into your blender. In medical jargon, this blob is called *chyme*, but we'll just stick with *blob*. Your stomach muscles contract to push the blob toward an opening located at its end, called the *pylorus*, which connects it to the next stop on your pizza's journey: your small intestine.

WHEN THINGS GO WRONG

Ever wonder why the bread and rolls served at restaurants are called "appetizers"? Remember how the pizza crust digests more quickly than the cheese and pepperoni? When you begin a meal with simple carbohydrates, such as white bread or pizza crust, which are rapidly broken down into sugars during the digestive process, they elevate the secretion of the hunger hormone *ghrelin*. Even though you've just stuffed yourself with bread, the secretion of ghrelin actually makes you feel hungrier. Restaurant owners may not have a degree in science, but they know from experience that appetizers entice you to order more food. That's good for the restaurateur, but bad for your hips and thighs.

WHEN YOU'RE LEAN FOR LIFE

In this book, you'll learn that eating high-quality protein and limiting—but not completely eliminating—carbohydrates is critical to getting your stomach and brain to work together to regulate your hunger hormones and reduce your appetite. As you'll see, the lean proteins you'll be eating on this program are converted into peptides, which play an important role in boosting satiety and preventing overeating.

YOUR SMALL BUT MIGHTY INTESTINE: YOUR BODY'S RECYCLING CENTER

The small intestine isn't small at all; in fact, it's about 20 feet long. The small intestine acts like a tollbooth, opening and closing the stomach's exit at its own discretion. To get past the tollbooth, the contents of your stomach must be sufficiently liquefied. If they're still too solid, your small intestine will close the exit and force the digesting food to make a U-turn back to your stomach for more mixing. Typically, it's the mashed-up carbs that get the green light first, with fats and proteins trailing behind because they take longer to dissolve.

Once the particles of your pizza make it into the small intestine, the breakdown continues and the preparations for the absorption of nutrients begin in earnest. But before your body can benefit from any of the nutrients in the foods you eat, it has to separate them from one another. Think of a recycling center, where people drop off cans, bottles, newspapers and other recyclable items. The facility can't dump everything it collects into the same machine, right? Glass materials must be sorted separately from the plastic, aluminum and paper before all of these materials can be processed into new glass bottles, plastic containers, aluminum cans and newspapers. If they weren't, you might cut yourself on glass while trying to read the newspaper, or your bottle of water might start leaking from all the paper mixed in with the plastic.

Your body is the ultimate recycling center, taking a bite of pizza and turning it into muscles, organs, brain cells and—of course—fat cells. To recycle your pizza, your small intestine must first sort out the proteins, carbs, fats, fiber, vitamins, minerals and water. For example, fats from the pepperoni, tomato sauce or crust are grouped with the fat from the cheese. Any protein that was in the cheese winds up with the protein from the pepperoni. And all the carbs huddle together in their own clique. No matter where they were originally on your slice of pizza, the nutrients are now deconstructed and separated into their most basic forms:

- Proteins are broken down into amino acids.

- Carbs are converted to sugars.

- Fats become fatty acids.

- Fiber from carbohydrates is separated out.

- Vitamins, minerals and water are sorted out and separated from all sources.

Helping your stomach and small intestine pulverize your bite of pizza are your liver and pancreas, which secrete a mixture of critical digestive juices that find their way into the small intestine.

- **Pancreas:** Your pancreas emits a number of enzymes to help process what used to be the cheese, pepperoni and crust of your bite of pizza. These include lipase for fats, *protease* for proteins and amylase for carbs, replacing the amylase first secreted by your salivary glands.

- **Liver:** Your liver produces *bile*, a thick green goo stored in the gallbladder until it is needed. When that bite of pizza shows up in your small intestine, the bile in the gallbladder is released into the small intestine, where it hunts out fat and dissolves it into a watery form. Once liquefied, the fat is digested by the lipase produced by the pancreas.

At this point, your pizza is completely unrecognizable. What began as a single slice is now divided into millions of microscopic molecular fragments. This pool of liquid is finally ready for the next leg of its journey: absorption into the 5 quarts of blood circulating in your bloodstream.

To help it on its way are millions of tiny finger-like structures called *villi* that line the intestinal wall and measure no more than 1 millimeter long. Your villi are covered with millions more *microvilli* that are 600 times smaller, and inside each villi are infinitesimally small capillaries. Think of all these miniature fingers "grabbing" the amino acids, sugars, fatty acids, vitamins, minerals and water and pushing them through the intestinal wall so they can be absorbed into the bloodstream.

Your miniature fingers don't wait for all nutrients to be equally broken down before transporting them into your blood. They grab onto whatever dissolves first, which are usually the carbohydrates that have been converted into sugars. Remember, carbohydrates from your pizza crust are pulverized and turned into sugars first. Amino acids from the pepperoni spend the most time in the intestine before being jettisoned into the bloodstream.

Unlike the sugars and amino acids, fatty acids from the meat and cheese take a detour before heading into the bloodstream. In the walls of the intestine, the fatty acids that have been broken down are reconstituted into triglycerides, cholesterol and other lipids. When these are pushed through the intestinal wall, they hitch a ride in your lymphatic system, which transports them to the bloodstream.

Once in your circulatory system, fats take a grand tour through many of the 60,000 miles of blood vessels that traverse your body. Some fats exit the bloodstream when they reach organs that need fats for optimal functioning, such as the brain. Regardless of their journey, the final destination is your liver, whose job it is to send any leftover lipids to your fat cells for storage.

The only thing that isn't processed by blood? Fiber, which has a different destination that we'll talk about later.

GUT CHECK—YOUR GUT'S SECURITY DETAIL

As your pizza makes its way through your gut, it also has to pass inspection by your gut's immune system. You may be surprised to discover that about 70 to 80 percent of your immune system is found within your gut. In particular, it's the lining of your intestines—a thin sheath that is only one cell-layer thick—that is in charge of protecting you from toxic materials, large chunks of undigested food, bacteria, viruses and more. Your intestinal lining also acts as a protective barrier, securing the contents of your gut from seeping out into your body, where it would be perceived as a foreign invader and attacked by immune cells throughout your body.

WHEN THINGS GO WRONG

Sometimes, your gut's immune system can become a little overprotective. In addition to destroying dangerous bacteria, viruses and toxic chemicals, it also attacks certain foods that come through your digestive tract. This may result in an intolerance to those foods—ever heard of *lactose intolerance*? Another potential problem is the breakdown of your intestinal barrier, which can occur as a result of intestinal infections or stress. This leads to something known as *leaky gut*, in which the contents of the gut can cross from inside the intestines to the body. The deeper problem is that the immune system sparks an inflammatory response not just within your gut but throughout your entire body. Later in this book, you'll discover much more about inflammation and how it impacts your weight.

WHEN YOU'RE LEAN FOR LIFE

By eating the foods recommended in this program and employing the strategies to help you stress less, you will begin to get your gut's immune system under control.

YOUR SECOND BRAIN

Closely monitoring all of this activity in your gut are some 200 million *neurons*—just like the ones you have in your brain—surrounding your intestine. With all of these neurons, your gut acts like a second brain in your body, a sort of on-site Mission Control that's communicating directly with the gray matter between your ears to keep it up to date on everything that's taking place down below. Your gut's Mission Control is constantly analyzing what's happening every millimeter of the way through your intestine and sending that information to your brain, allowing it to regulate the process.

For example, the arrival of protein into your intestine sparks a flurry of communication between your second brain and your big brain upstairs. This results in the secretion of the hormone cholecystokinin (CCK), which aids in the assimilation of amino acids and helps switch off hunger. It also triggers an increase in glucose in the *portal vein*, the main vein that carries blood from the stomach and intestines to the liver. This increase in glucose here helps fight hunger for hours.

WHEN THINGS GO WRONG

Unfortunately, your second brain doesn't always communicate effectively with the gray matter inside your head. Overeating on a regular basis or eating too many of the wrong kinds of food can slow or disrupt the messaging process. In some cases, your big brain becomes desensitized to the constant messaging and ignores your second brain. And if for any reason, your big brain doesn't get or doesn't acknowledge the message that you just ate a slice of filling pepperoni pizza, you're likely to eat another, and another, and even another.

WHEN YOU'RE LEAN FOR LIFE

By eating the specific foods recommended in this program, you can re-establish the lines of communication between your second brain and your big brain to prevent overeating.

BUG ME!

Who knew that on its fantastic voyage throughout your digestive system, your bite of pizza would meet up with a massive army of bugs? That's right: occupying your intestines are more than 100 trillion bugs called *microflora*. In fact, there are so many of these bacteria living in your gut that they outnumber your body's cells 10 to 1! Is this a problem? Just the opposite. In healthy people, these critters are beneficial to the digestive process, helping convert carbs into sugars and proteins into amino acids. Scientists have already identified more than 1,000 types of bacteria in the digestive system. Throughout this book, you'll discover much more about your gut microflora, the role they play in your weight, and what you can do to make sure you've got a healthy balance of microflora.

It's important to understand that the bugs in your gut aren't necessarily working *for* you. They are independent, living beings that are primarily interested in their own survival and reproduction. These bugs communicate with your brain and body to encourage you to consume the foods that will help them flourish.

WHEN THINGS GO WRONG

In some people, the digestive system has been invaded by bands of trouble-making bugs. Like the beneficial bugs in your gut, these bad guys also want to proliferate.

They influence your brain and body to eat the foods—such as refined carbs and sugar—that will allow them to multiply. When there are too many harmful bacteria in your gut, it can reinforce unhealthy eating habits, wreak havoc with digestion and cause your weight to soar.

Just as the bacteria in your gut can influence what you want to eat, the foods you eat have a significant impact on the makeup of the bug colonies in your gut. Consuming too many foods high in sugar or refined carbohydrates can wipe out many of the beneficial bugs in your digestive tract, promote the growth of harmful gut bacteria and lead to problems. When the composition of your gut microflora is off balance, it is suspected to play a role in food cravings, inflammation, insulin resistance and problems burning calories—all of which make it so much harder for you to lose weight.

WHEN YOU'RE LEAN FOR LIFE
In this book you'll learn what foods promote the growth of bugs that not only improve digestion but also may make it easier for you to win the battle of the bulge.

LEAVE IT TO YOUR LIVER
All that nutrient-infused blood eventually heads to your liver, which quickly weeds out harmful substances and then dictates where the various nutrients will go in your body. Like a construction foreman, your liver tells all the incoming workers where to go and what they'll be doing:

- *Sugars, head to the cells to provide energy.*

- *Amino acids, find your way to the muscles, organs and tissues, and start regenerating cells and making repairs.*

- *Fatty acids, go directly to the fat cells and wait there until I say otherwise.*

WHEN THINGS GO WRONG
If you've eaten too many slices of pizza, your liver may tell the surplus of sugars to change into fatty acids and join the crew heading for your fat cells. When you've spent years eating too many slices of pizza, your fat cells swell from taking in so many fatty acids, and it eventually shows up on your body in the form of a spare tire, muffin top, love handles, saddlebags or some other unwanted flab. If your fat cells become full and can't hold any more, your liver tells any excess sugars and fatty acids to just hang tight right there in the liver in a sort of holding pattern. This leads to a fatty liver (which you'll learn more about on Day 18 in chapter 6).

Unfortunately, when you accumulate too much fat, it also causes your brain and body to "forget" how to burn fat. How can your body forget something so basic? Think back to when you took high school French or any other foreign language. If you paid attention in class, you probably got to the point where you could have a decent conversation *en français*. But if you never used your French after graduation, you probably forgot most of it. Then 10 years later, if you took a trip to Paris, your French would be rusty and you'd probably have trouble remembering anything more than the most rudimentary phrases, like *Bonjour, ça va?* After a few days in the City of Lights, however, some of your high school French would start coming back to you, and by the end of your trip you could be *parlez-vous*-ing with ease. Similarly, if your body has been fueling itself primarily with glucose, it will likely take a few days or even a couple of weeks for it to remember how to tap into your fat cells for fuel.

WHEN YOU'RE LEAN FOR LIFE

On this program, you'll learn which foods and which portions will keep your liver sending nutrients to their proper destinations so that you can feel great and stay lean. Even better, following this program will help your fat cells remember how to burn fat and shrink in size. This is very important because fat cells don't die! They can only change their size. Research shows that this program helps shrink the size of fat cells twice as much as other diets. Shrinking your fat cells is the only way to shrink your waistline.

YOUR LARGE INTESTINE: STUCK WITH THE LEFTOVERS

Now let's go back to the fiber that didn't get absorbed into your bloodstream. Whereas other nutrients are absorbed into the bloodstream in your small intestine, fiber heads into your large intestine for further processing. The last remains of your pizza camp out in the part of the large intestine called the colon for a day or two, which is how long it takes to traverse the 5 feet to the rectum. This is your body's last chance to harvest any remaining nutrients or water from your pizza.

Dozens of species of bacteria inhabit your large intestine, and they feed off the fibrous material that passes through. To assimilate the dietary fiber, these bacteria produce enzymes such as hydrogen and methane, which your body rejects by passing gas. Your colon acts like a trash compactor, compressing the dry leftovers as they move along until they form a solid stool. After a visit to the restroom, your slice of pizza's amazing journey comes to an end with a flush.

WHEN THINGS GO WRONG

Eating too much pizza or too much of the wrong kinds of food can result in a variety of uncomfortable, embarrassing digestive woes.

WHEN YOU'RE LEAN FOR LIFE

With the tips and tactics revealed in the pages of this book, you can keep your digestive system moving smoothly so you can avoid constipation and other types of digestive distress.

THE BRAIN-BODY-GUT COMMUNICATION SYSTEM

As you've followed the journey of your slice of pizza, you've seen that your brain, body and gut are supposed to communicate and cooperate in an effort to keep you lean. It's as if your brain, body and gut are all using smart phones to send and receive messages to and from each other.

WHEN THINGS GO WRONG

Let's look more closely at the brain-body-gut communications system and what happens when it goes on the fritz. If you've ever had a day when your smart phone stopped working and you couldn't send or receive emails or text messages, you know that you can't get anything done right. That's what it's like in your body, too. When you're overweight, your brain, body and gut stop working together to keep information flowing smoothly. Instead, they behave more like three self-absorbed "neighbors" living inside your body, jockeying for attention. And just like neighbors anywhere, all three are interested in one thing and one thing only: their own needs. Your brain, body and gut are all primarily concerned with their own survival.

When you're carrying too much weight, the text messages they send out aren't supportive and encouraging. Don't expect your bad gut microflora to text: *Hey brain, good job saying no to that extra slice of pizza so it doesn't kill off more of the good microflora down here. Way to go! Let's work together to keep the pizza intake down and boost the veggie intake next time. Okay?* Instead, if your gut has been overrun by harmful microflora, it is more likely to text: *OMG, that pizza was soooo good! I can't get enough of that dough. Tell that mouth to get some more down here, pronto!*

Meanwhile, your liver is overrun with a glut of sugar from all the carbohydrates in that dough, and it's texting your brain: *Unable to keep up with all this sugar. If it keeps coming in, I'll have to store it here until I can figure out where to send it.*

And what's your brain doing with all the conflicting messages it's receiving? That depends. Sometimes it's a matter of who's screaming—or texting—the loudest. If the gut has too much harmful microflora, it is likely to be bellowing repeatedly for more carbs and more sugar while the liver more quietly goes about its business trying to cope with the flood of sugars. In other instances, the brain may become desensitized to all the incoming messages, and it no longer "listens" to the body or gut. In addition, remember that, like your bodily organs and your gut microflora, your brain has its own desires. Through a complex and very powerful reward system, which you'll learn more about later, the brain derives pleasure from eating and in particular from highly palatable foods.

In some people, the brain is so intent on getting what it wants that it acts without any consideration for the rest of your body. It may demand certain foods or quantities of food that give it pleasure but that damage your gut, liver and pancreas. It's similar to the way people continue to smoke in spite of knowing all the health risks it presents. In this scenario, the brain basically shuts off communication with its neighbors, which is really bad news.

Imagine all those text messages efficiently traveling through your body, telling all of your systems how best to serve you, and then your brain sending out only one message: *No Service.* The messages your digestive system is trying to send to your brain—*Trying to digest an entire pint of ice cream down here. Can't handle all this fat and sugar. Don't send any more.*—are blocked, which means your brain never registers that you just chowed down, and so you eat another pint, and maybe even another. This breakdown in communication helps explain why you may have developed some of the habits that can make you fat and keep you fat.

WHEN YOU'RE LEAN FOR LIFE

Lean for Life is a comprehensive program designed to get your brain-body-gut team—the "BBG gang"—working and communicating effectively again so you can stop gaining weight and start getting leaner.

PRESTO CHANGE-O! YOUR SLICE OF PIZZA HAS TURNED INTO A SPARE TIRE

As you can clearly see, that slice of pizza didn't turn into a spare tire by magic. By taking a look inside your body, it's easy to understand that when you eat too many slices of pizza—or too much of any fat-promoting foods—your brain, body and gut can conspire to transform them into a spare tire, muffin top, saddlebags, or all of the above. Once your brain, body and gut—the "BBG gang"—start plotting together to store excess fat, they can become locked in conspiracy mode and make you a slave to the habits that can supersize you.

With so many complex processes at work here, it becomes clear why there is no magic bullet or magic pill for weight loss. It's just not that simple. The good news is that Lean for Life is a comprehensive program designed to outsmart your biology and get your brain, body and gut working for you. Throughout this book, you'll learn much more about the various biological processes described here—as well as the many psychological, behavioral and environmental factors contributing to weight gain—and you'll discover specific actions you can take to reverse the problems so you can lose weight quickly and keep it off, not just for a month but for life. With the easy-to-follow blueprint in this book, you can lose up to 20 pounds in 28 days while you heal your gut, reprogram your appetite, rewire your brain, calm cravings and shrink your fat cells.

With all these benefits in mind, are you ready to start your Lean for Life adventure?

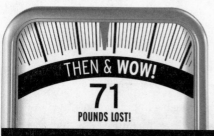

THEN & **WOW!**

71
POUNDS LOST!

Kristina Kampen

AGE
21

OCCUPATION
Student

HEIGHT
5'7"

CURRENT WEIGHT
135

LARGEST SIZE
16

CURRENT SIZE
4

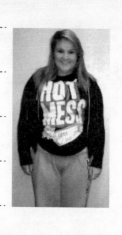

The extra weight I carried around all those years really weighed me down—literally and figuratively. I now know what it feels like to be happy in my own skin and to have a sense of optimism about my life and my future.

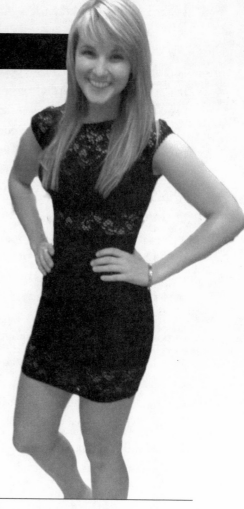

TURNING POINT: When I gained 40 pounds during my freshman year of college, I knew things had to change. I didn't like the person I had become. I would be mean to other girls just because I was jealous of them. I was miserable, bitter and out of control. My mom had lost 35 pounds on the Lean for Life program two years earlier, so I knew it worked.

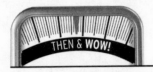

LOSSES AND GAINS: When you start making big improvements in your life, it can sometimes make the people around you uncomfortable. Not everyone wanted to see me succeed. You quickly learn who your real friends are. Some people were really unsupportive of my weight loss and tried to sabotage my success by tempting me into eating foods that weren't on my program or going to fast-food places where making healthy choices was much tougher. It was sort of like the "buddy system" in reverse! Fortunately, my parents and lots of other friends were supportive, and that gave me the courage and strength to stay focused and to follow through.

WHO'S THAT GIRL? I started my Lean for Life program during the last half of my freshman year in college. When I returned for my sophomore year, a guy came up to me and asked if I was a new student. I couldn't believe it. We had sat next to each other for an entire semester, but he didn't recognize me. He wasn't the only one. There were a lot of people who told me I seemed like a different person—and they were right! Not only did I look different, but I also grew up a lot as a result of taking control and responsibility for my health and my appearance.

MAKING THE CONNECTION: Once I began more fully appreciating the link between my brain, my body and even my gut—and how they're so interconnected—I became much more conscious of my behavior, my thoughts and my actions. What we eat, what we do and what we think all matters.

BIG CHANGES: I relate to the world very differently since I've gotten down to a healthy weight. My attitude and outlook are so much more upbeat.

RETRAIN YOUR BRAIN, BODY AND GUT TO THINK AND ACT LEAN

When the "BBG gang" has enslaved you to the habits that can cause weight gain, you need to retrain your brain, body and gut to think and act lean. The Lean for Life program will help you do it. With this program, you'll learn how to "leanify" your eating habits, daily routines and thought patterns so you can outsmart your brain, body and gut. Replacing old, unhealthy habits with lean habits is the key to becoming Lean for Life. If you're ready to get started, you're probably wondering: *So what do I eat?*

After more than 15 million patient visits to our Lindora Clinics, we know to expect this question from new patients. This innocent query reveals one of the most common reasons why so many diets fail—losing weight and maintaining that weight loss isn't *only* about food. If it were as simple as knowing *what* to eat, then everybody could lose weight and keep it off. We know that eating the right foods at the right times in the right quantities is a key component to getting and staying lean, but we also understand that there are many other physiological, psychological, behavioral and environmental factors at play. To achieve rapid weight loss and keep it off, all of these factors must be addressed.

That's why the Lean for Life program is one part biology modification— which we refer to as BioMod—and one part behavior modification—which we refer to as behavior mod. What does that mean? It means that this program's eating plan and success strategies are designed to outsmart your biology to get your brain, body and gut working for you instead of against you. That's the BioMod. It also means that this is a comprehensive lifestyle program that goes beyond traditional food plans to help you transform your thinking habits, your daily routines and your life. That's the behavior mod. The results? Rapid weight loss and a leaner, healthier body.

Based on more than 40 years of hands-on experience working with hundreds of thousands of people just like you, we know that sticking with a diet plan isn't easy. That's why Lean for Life holds your hand throughout your program to help you deal with the biological stumbling blocks, emotional issues, mental hurdles and everyday obstacles that typically sabotage weight loss and contribute to weight gain. We'll be with you every step of the way, offering helpful tips and techniques *to help you succeed on your program.* This will help you stick with your plan so you can reach your ideal lean weight and maintain your new weight. As Dr. Stamper says, "It's entirely within your power to rethink, reprogram and redefine the role food plays in your life. The Lean for Life program will show you how."

How does the program work? The Lean for Life program is simple, and it boils down to four phases, as shown in "The New Lean for Life Overview."

1. The Prep
2. Rapid Weight Loss
3. Metabolic Adjustment
4. Metabolic Equilibrium

PHASE 1: THE PREP

The Prep is a three-day crash course to prepare your brain, body and gut for maximum results. You'll find instructions for this phase in chapter 3.

PHASE 2: RAPID WEIGHT LOSS

Phase 2 of the Lean for Life program, Rapid Weight Loss, is the heart of this book—that's when you'll really see the pounds drop off. In chapters 4 through 7, we provide the details on what to eat and the basics of what you'll be doing during the all-important Rapid Weight Loss phase so you can be prepared. We give you all the tools you need as you do the program day by day.

During Rapid Weight Loss, you'll be following Lean for Life's smart carb eating plan, which has been refined over more than 40 years and has already helped hundreds of thousands of patients lose more than 15 million pounds.

THE NEW LEAN FOR LIFE OVERVIEW

PHASE 1–THE PREP: 3 DAYS

The Prep primes your brain, body and gut for Rapid Weight Loss.

PHASE 2–RAPID WEIGHT LOSS: 1 CYCLE = 28 DAYS

Rapid Weight Loss helps you achieve dietary ketosis to accelerate fat burning and shrink your fat cells. You may do a *maximum* of two cycles of Rapid Weight Loss in a row.

Days 1-3	Protein Days
Days 4-7	Menu Days
Day 8	Protein Day
Days 9-14	Menu Days
Day 15	Protein Day
Days 16-21	Menu Days
Day 22	Protein Day
Days 23-28	Menu Days

PHASE 3–METABOLIC ADJUSTMENT: 1 CYCLE = 14 DAYS

Metabolic Adjustment corrects for the decrease in resting metabolic rate that occurs with calorie restriction. The goal is to gradually increase calorie intake *without gaining weight*.

Day 1	Protein Day
Days 2-3	Metabolic Adjustment, Level 1
Days 4-7	Metabolic Adjustment, Level 2
Day 8	Protein Day
Days 9-14	Metabolic Adjustment, Level 3

After successfully completing Metabolic Adjustment, you have two options. If you want to lose more weight, begin another Rapid Weight Loss cycle followed by another Metabolic Adjustment period. If you've achieved your ideal lean weight, proceed to Metabolic Equilibrium.

PHASE 4–METABOLIC EQUILIBRIUM

Metabolic Equilibrium is a lifestyle program intended to keep you Lean for Life. To keep on track, continue doing one Protein Day per week for life.

Alternating between Protein Days and Menu Days, our plan centers on a moderate protein, low-calorie, smart-carb (see "Smart Carbs That Count" on page 23 for more on this), low-fat structured eating plan that is designed to achieve the beneficial state of dietary ketosis.

Ketosis simply means that the body is burning fat as fuel, which causes fat cells to shrink in size. Ketosis occurs whenever you significantly limit your intake of carbohydrates, which are the body's primary source of energy. When your body has used up all of its energy stores from carbohydrates, it switches

Dr. Stamper Says

THE SIX ESSENTIALS

Dr. Stamper's Six Essentials are powerful, fundamental truths that are the cornerstones of the Lean for Life program. They will guide you through your program and help you achieve your rapid weight loss. We have found that the people who are the most successful on this program are the ones who have learned to integrate Dr. Stamper's Six Essentials into their daily lives. "I call them the Six Essentials," Dr. Stamper explains, "because I'm convinced that once you understand these concepts and master them, you'll never again need to diet. You will truly *be* Lean for Life."

1. Make it your goal to *learn* to be Lean for Life.

2. Learn to control cravings.

3. Your level of interest and enthusiasm will determine your level of success.

4. Learn to recognize and eliminate your defensive barriers.

5. Learn to use relaxation techniques and stress less.

6. Maintain healthy behaviors for lasting success.

Throughout this book, we'll introduce you to the Six Essentials one at a time.

to its alternate fuel source—fat. Lean for Life uses the power of ketosis to help you burn fat, shrink your fat cells and get leaner.

Dietary ketosis has remained the foundation of this phase of the program for more than 40 years not only because it produces excellent weight-loss results, but also because it provides a host of other benefits that make it easier to stick with the program. You'll discover much more about these benefits throughout the book, but here is a sneak peek at some of the things ketosis and this eating plan can do to help you get leaner on this program:

- Shrink fat cells.
- Accelerate weight loss.
- Increase satiety and reduce hunger.
- Reduce cravings.
- Increase physical and mental energy.
- Enhance moods.
- Decrease irritability.
- Reduce feelings of depression.
- Boost motivation.
- Reduce gut inflammation.

As you can see, dietary ketosis can be one of your greatest allies in your battle against the bulge. *Note: A ketogenic diet is not recommended for type 1 insulin-dependent diabetics, pregnant or nursing mothers, or people with serious liver or kidney disease. If you have any concerns or questions, consult your physician before beginning this program.*

HOW DO YOU KNOW IF YOU'RE IN KETOSIS?

When you burn a larger amount of fat than is immediately needed for energy, the excess ketones are eliminated in the urine. During Rapid Weight Loss, you'll be monitoring your urine every morning using a ketone-measuring strip, also known as a ketostick—or what we refer to as Fat-Burning Indicators. When significant levels of ketones are detected, a reactive pad on the end of the ketostick changes color, ranging from pink to purple. This indicates that you're in ketosis. If the ketostick doesn't change color, it means you're not in ketosis.

The Inside Story from Dr. Allouche

FOOD AS FUEL

THE POWER OF PROTEIN

Why is protein so important in helping you get leaner? Protein is found in every single cell in your body, including in your bones, muscles, organs, glands and skin. It is also involved in the production of hormones, enzymes and your immune system, and it is responsible for building, maintaining and repairing tissues. There is so much protein in the human body that it accounts for 16 percent of body weight in lean individuals.

When protein is digested, it is broken down into amino acids, which are the building blocks for proteins in your body. Your body produces some of the amino acids that are critical to optimal health on its own, but there are eight amino acids, called the essential amino acids, that you can get only through food. The problem is that your body can't store amino acids the way it stores fat. This means you must consume proteins containing all of the essential amino acids every day. If you don't, it can weaken your immune system, hamper your body's ability to repair muscle tissue, and subsequently, lower your metabolism. High protein-efficiency ratio (PER) proteins, such as the ones you'll be consuming on this program, provide the highest content of amino acids for optimal benefit.

Increasing your protein consumption, as you'll be doing on this program, strengthens your immune system, facilitates muscle repair and boosts metabolism. In addition, it helps keep hunger at bay. At Lindora and in my own practice, we've long known that protein helps suppress our patients' appetites, but the latest satiety science is just now beginning to reveal some of the many reasons why.

Protein Alone Discourages Overeating. Sure, most of us look forward to having turkey on Thanksgiving, but imagine if your entire holiday meal consisted of nothing but the turkey—no green beans, no stuffing, no sweet potatoes with marshmallows, and no pumpkin pie for dessert. You probably wouldn't overindulge the way you typically do.

It Takes Longer to Digest Protein Than Any Other Nutrient. You saw this during the amazing journey of that slice of pizza in chapter 1. In fact, it requires so much effort to digest protein that for every 100 calories of protein you consume, your body is burning 25 calories just to digest it.

Eating Protein Reduces Levels of the Hunger Hormone Ghrelin. When levels of ghrelin, which is released by the stomach, are high, it sends messages to the brain saying, *I'm hungry.* When levels are low, it reduces your appetite. Some studies show that ghrelin levels are suppressed for up to three hours after a protein-rich meal. You'll discover much more about your appetite hormones in upcoming chapters.

Protein Consumption Triggers the Release of the Digestive Hormone CCK. When the gut releases CCK, it reduces hunger.

Certain Peptides Found in Proteins Increase Satiety. Through my research, I have identified certain peptides, which are molecules found in proteins, that set in motion a series of signals that fend off hunger. You'll learn more about these peptides throughout the book.

To quickly recap, eating adequate amounts of lean protein as you'll be doing during Rapid Weight Loss offers a variety of weight-loss benefits. The right amounts of protein in your diet:

- Increase satiety.
- Reduce hunger.
- Reduce cravings.
- Maintain lean muscle mass to boost metabolism.

SMART CARBS THAT COUNT

While you're on this program, you'll be taking our smart-carb approach and counting carbohydrates. As you saw in the amazing journey of that slice of pizza in chapter 1, eating too many carbs can lead to a breakdown in communication among your brain, body and gut and can result in excess fat storage, cravings and ultimately a spare tire. In terms of digestion, carbs are classified as either simple or complex, depending on their molecular makeup.

Simple carbs, also known as refined carbs, are made up of only one or two glucose molecules and race through your digestive system quickly, causing a rapid and sharp rise in your blood sugar levels and consequently your insulin levels. With little to no nutritional value, simple carbs get absorbed into the bloodstream and shuttled to the liver, which usually sends them to be stored as fat in your fat cells. Foods that contain simple carbs include table sugar, honey, sodas, cakes, candy, fruit, fruit juice, jams, milk, yogurt, many breakfast cereals and of course the white flour crust of your pizza.

Complex carbs are made up of three or more glucose molecules that are linked together to form a chain. Your digestive system has to work hard to un-link that chain, so these carbs spend more time on their incredible journey through your body. Because they take longer to be digested and absorbed, they don't have the same effect on blood sugar and insulin levels as simple carbs. Complex carbs are found in vegetables, whole grains and legumes, which are packed with vitamins and minerals. These carbs also contain varying amounts of fiber, which add bulk to your diet. Within complex carbs, there are two types of fiber: soluble and insoluble.

- **Soluble fiber:** As it is digested, soluble fiber attracts water and morphs into a gel-like substance that slows digestion to increase satiety. One type of soluble fiber called *inulin* also acts as a "prebiotic," which means that it stimulates the growth of beneficial bacteria in your intestine. Inulin also improves absorption of vitamins and minerals and helps prevent constipation. Look for inulin in fiber supplements and Lean for Life products.

- **Insoluble fiber:** This type of fiber helps speed food through your digestive system and adds bulk to your stool. The bugs in your gut have to work very hard to process this type of fiber, which may produce gas.

THE CARB-SUGAR CONNECTION

When digested, both simple and complex carbs are converted into sugars. For every 100 calories of carbs consumed, your body burns 10 calories to complete this process. In a normal meal, 70 percent of sugars are absorbed into the bloodstream and burned off as energy within about six hours. The remaining 30 percent are transformed into triglycerides by your adipose tissue and stored in your fat cells. When you eat too many carbohydrates of any kind, more of them are transformed into triglycerides and stored in your fat cells.

Every time you eat carbs, it raises your blood sugar and triggers the secretion of insulin from the pancreas. When you habitually overdo it on carbs, you wear out your pancreas and your body becomes less sensitive to the insulin it releases. This is called insulin resistance, and it can lead to type 2 diabetes. (See more on insulin resistance on Day 15 in chapter 6.)

CARBS AND THE GLYCEMIC INDEX

The Glycemic Index (GI) rates carbohydrates based on their effect on blood sugar levels and insulin levels. The higher the GI ranking, the higher the blood sugar levels will be, causing more insulin produced, which is bad news for your waistline. Too much sugar being dumped rapidly into your bloodstream leads to too much insulin and ultimately, too much sugar being stored in your fat cells. Sugars and refined carbs, such as those in pizza crust, rank high on the GI and cause you to pack on unwanted pounds.

On the other hand, complex carbs that rank lower on the GI, such as whole grains and non-starchy vegetables, are wrapped in fiber, so it takes longer for your gut microflora to separate the sugar from the fiber. This slows the absorption of these sugars and reduces the impact on blood sugar and insulin levels. Less insulin results in less sugar being stored in your fat cells.

During the Rapid Weight Loss phase, it is best to focus the majority of your meals on foods that are low GI (below 55) to keep you feeling full, reduce cravings, and produce the ideal conditions for burning fat and shrinking fat cells. Here's a quick look at where some foods rank. For a more complete list, see the "Glycemic Index Chart" in Appendix C.

- **High-GI carbs (70 and over),** which include frozen yogurt, hard candy, rice cakes, and baked potatoes, cause insulin and blood sugar levels to spike rapidly. The rise in insulin encourages fat storing and prevents fat burning. Not only that, about an hour after eating a high-GI meal, your blood sugar level crashes, leaving you feeling sleepy, sluggish and craving more simple carbs. And the cycle starts all over again.

- **Moderate-GI carbs (55 to 69),** such as quinoa, bananas, and grapes, cause a moderate rise in insulin and blood sugar levels.

- **Low-GI carbs (below 55)** include non-starchy vegetables, apples, cherries, oranges, oatmeal (steel cut or slow cooking), yogurt (nonfat, plain), and skim milk and cause a lower rise in insulin and blood sugar levels, which creates more favorable fat-burning conditions in your body. Plus, there's no crash after you eat, so you feel full longer and reduce cravings. The Lean for Life program is considered a low-glycemic program that helps balance blood sugar and insulin levels so you can start shrinking your fat cells and shrinking your waistline.

GET YOUR FATS STRAIGHT

You may feel like you're at war with the fat on your body, but did you know that dietary fat supports brain health, cardiovascular function and your immune system? Fats also act as transporters to help your body absorb a number of important vitamins, including vitamins A, D, E and K. But not all fats are created equal.

"GREEN-LIGHT" FATS

Healthy fats include monounsaturated fats (MUFAs) and polyunsaturated fats (PUFAs). Found in olive oil, MUFAs are potentially beneficial to your health. Research shows that they can improve cholesterol levels, enhance insulin sensitivity and help stabilize blood sugar levels. MUFAs have also been linked to a decrease in inflammation and a reduction in belly fat.

PUFAs contain essential fatty acids known as omega-3 and omega-6 fatty acids. Your body needs these fats for a variety of important functions, but it doesn't produce enough of them on its own, so you need to get these fats in your diet. Like MUFAs, PUFAs are associated with improved heart health, lower blood pressure levels, decreased inflammation and less belly fat.

The "Lean Foods" list at the end of this chapter indicates which foods are high in health-promoting omega-3 fatty acids.

"YELLOW-LIGHT" FATS

Saturated fats are found primarily in animal food sources, such as meats, cheese and butter, as well as in some plant oils, such as palm oil and coconut oil. In recent years, saturated fats have gotten a lot of bad press. Because of this, it may be surprising to learn that these fats play a vital role in many physiological processes, including building cell membranes and producing healthy hormones. You need to exercise some caution though, because only a small amount of these fats are needed. When consumed in excess, saturated fats may be harmful to your health. Eating too many saturated fats may raise total cholesterol levels, including levels of low-density lipoprotein (LDL), the bad type of cholesterol that is linked to cardiovascular disease.

"RED-LIGHT" FATS

The worst type of fats for your waistline and for your health are called trans fats. Food manufacturers use partial hydrogenation to convert unsaturated fats into trans fats to increase the shelf life of packaged foods, such as crackers, cookies and other baked goods. These dangerous "Frankenfats" raise LDL, the bad cholesterol, levels and lower levels of high-density lipoprotein (HDL), the good cholesterol, raising the risk for heart disease.

No matter which types of fat you consume, remember that they are all high in calories—9 calories per gram. And remember that it takes very little effort for your body to convert those fats into the fatty acids that get stored in your fat cells. In fact, for every 100 calories of fats you consume, your body burns only 1 meager calorie to digest' it.

PROTEIN DAYS

Rapid Weight Loss begins with three Protein Days that place an emphasis on protein intake while restricting—but not eliminating—carbohydrates. Your Protein Days play a pivotal role in your journey to becoming Lean for Life— jump-starting rapid weight loss and gently guiding your body into dietary ketosis. After the first week of the Rapid Weight Loss phase, you'll continue doing one Protein Day per week.

On your Protein Days, eat high-quality proteins. Think salmon, chicken or turkey breast, lean beef, eggs or egg whites, tofu and low-fat cottage cheese—all foods you can easily find in any grocery store or restaurant. Don't have time to cook or don't enjoy spending time in the kitchen? Don't worry: you have options. At our Lindora Clinics, we have discovered that our patients enjoy more rapid and sustained weight loss when our program allows them to rely on convenience foods as they do when they aren't "on a diet." If you prefer the convenience of ready-made meals and grab-and-go snacks, feel free to take advantage of the Lean for Life protein bars, soups, cookies, pancakes, shakes, puddings, chips and other snacks that contain special proteins that increase satiety and accelerate weight loss. If you'd prefer to grab something at your local grocery store, that's okay, too. Just be sure to check the protein snack guidelines that follow to make the best choices when shopping.

Because so many of our patients rely on these convenience foods, all of the menu plans in this book offer the option of making food or enjoying prepared foods and snacks. Feel free to mix and match. It's entirely up to you.

WHAT TO EAT ON YOUR PROTEIN DAYS

On your Protein Days, follow these guidelines:

- **Eat a protein serving every two to two and a half hours.** To control hunger, maintain energy and boost metabolism, do not go more than two and a half hours without having a protein serving. For example, if you have breakfast at 7:00 a.m., you may have a morning snack at 9:00 a.m., a late-morning snack at 11:00 a.m., lunch at 1:00 p.m., an afternoon snack at 3:00 p.m., a late-afternoon snack at 5:00 p.m., dinner at 7:00 p.m., and an evening snack at 9:00 p.m. Depending on your current weight and your activity level, you may need more—or fewer—protein servings. As a rule, consume a *minimum* of six protein servings per day on your Protein Days. Serving sizes are indicated on the "Lean Foods" list at the end of the chapter.

- **Choose high protein-efficiency ratio (PER) proteins.** If you want the best results, choose proteins that have a high PER. High PER proteins contain the greatest amounts of certain key nutrients that are involved in reducing the desire to eat, helping the brain recognize signals of hunger and satiety, and increasing fat metabolism. For the highest-quality proteins, stick with those listed on the "Lean Foods" list and any of the Lean for Life protein products, which you can read more about in Appendix B.

View Lean for Life high PER protein products.

- **Limit carbohydrate intake to approximately 50 to 80 grams per day.** Do not eat any fruits or vegetables, or any other foods that are not on the "Lean Foods" protein list. The 50 to 80 grams of carbohydrates you will be consuming on these days must come solely from the recommended proteins. You'll see that some of the protein foods contain higher amounts of carbohydrates than others. For example, low-fat and nonfat cottage cheese and yogurt have more carbs than chicken or fish. Choose your proteins accordingly. For your first two initial Protein Days, aim for the higher range of carbs (80 grams). If you're not in ketosis by the morning of Day 3, reduce your carb intake to the lower range.

- **Know what to look for in store-bought protein snacks.** Look for protein bars with at least 10 grams of protein (15 grams is even better!), no more than 200 calories (160 calories is better!), less than 20 grams of total carbs, and no more than 5 or 6 grams of fat. Carefully check the total carbs content to be sure you don't exceed 50 to 80 grams of carbs for the day. A few brands that meet these parameters include Pure Protein bars and Met-Rx Minis (33-gram size).

You can see how these guidelines come together in the "Sample Protein Day Menu."

SAMPLE PROTEIN DAY MENU

BREAKFAST

1 egg or 2 egg whites
OR
1 Lean for Life pancake

MORNING SNACK

2 ounces fat-free cheese
OR
1 ounce Lean for Life Salted Soy Nuts

LATE-MORNING SNACK (OPTIONAL, IF HUNGRY)

½ cup plain, nonfat yogurt
OR
1 Lean for Life Island Fruit Smoothie Shake Mix

LUNCH

2½ ounces water-packed tuna
OR
1 Lean for Life Homestyle Chicken Soup with Noodles

continued

SAMPLE PROTEIN DAY MENU

AFTERNOON SNACK

4 ounces low-fat cottage cheese

OR

1 Lean for Life Peanut Butter Crunch bar

LATE-AFTERNOON SNACK (OPTIONAL, IF HUNGRY)

3 1/2 ounces shrimp

OR

1 Lean for Life Sour Cream & Onion Crunch O's

DINNER

3 1/2 ounces chicken or turkey breast

OR

1 Lean for Life Savory Beef Soup with Vegetables

EVENING SNACK

2 1/2 ounces lean/fat-free cold cuts

OR

1 Lean for Life Cinnamon Oatmeal Raisin bar (heat it in the microwave
for 10 seconds—it might remind you of apple cobbler)

MENU DAYS

After completing your initial Protein Days, you'll transition to your Menu Days
for the remainder of the first week. On subsequent weeks, you'll do one Protein
Day per week followed by six Menu Days. On Menu Days, there's no need to
track protein grams, but you will need to continue maintaining your carbohydrate intake at 50 to 80 grams per day. *Before you eat anything on your Menu
Days, know how many carbs it contains.* This ensures that you will remain in the
fat cell–shrinking state of ketosis.

On Menu Days, you'll be eating three meals plus three high PER protein
snacks a day. You'll be able to choose from more than 100 delicious foods on
the "Lean Foods" list, including high-quality proteins, non-starchy vegetables,
fruits, whole grains and unlimited greens. You may substitute high PER protein

products for whole-food proteins, but this is the only substitution allowed. Understand that the foods on these lists as well as the structure of the eating plan have been revised and refined over more than 40 years based on the latest nutritional science and our clinical experience with hundreds of thousands of patients. They have been carefully chosen for their ability to enhance satiety, reduce cravings, spark weight loss, shrink fat cells and ensure ketosis. For this reason, you are encouraged to resist the temptation to modify the food choices or the structure of the eating plans.

View more detailed food lists.

WHAT TO EAT ON YOUR MENU DAYS

On your Menu Days, follow these guidelines:

- **Eat three meals and three high PER protein snacks per day.** Follow the "Menu Days Menu Plan" on page 33 and choose your foods from the "Lean Foods" list at the end of the chapter. You'll be eating meals for your breakfast, lunch and dinner in addition to one protein snack each at mid-morning, mid-afternoon and after dinner. Some people may need more than three protein snacks a day to control hunger and maintain energy, especially if physically active.

- **Do not go more than two and a half hours without eating and allow approximately four to five hours between meals.** For example, if you have breakfast at 8:00 a.m., have a high PER protein snack by 10:30 a.m., lunch by 1:00 p.m., a protein snack by 3:30 p.m., dinner by 6:00 p.m. and a final protein snack no later than 8:30 p.m.

- **Do not combine meals or "save" foods to eat at another time.** The meals are structured to provide an appropriate balance of protein, carbs and total calories to maintain ketosis, promote optimal weight loss and reduce cravings. In addition, the Menu Days are structured to help you develop intentional eating habits that will help you control your weight for life.

- **Do not skip meals or eat less food.** Skipping meals or eating less than is recommended may lower your metabolism, compromise your nutritional status and trigger cravings.

- **Prepare foods without the use of oils or fats.** Use a light coating of nonstick cooking spray instead, with one exception. You may use up to 1 teaspoon per day (2 tablespoons per week) of olive, flaxseed, canola or walnut oil when cooking or as a salad dressing, as all of these oils are rich in essential fatty acids that serve important metabolic roles and are important for brain health. Do not exceed this amount.

- **Accurately weigh and measure all servings.** Use a food scale and measuring cups and spoons to make sure you are eating the proper serving sizes. Weigh servings after cooking, and when using measuring cups and spoons, be sure to use "level" measurements to ensure accuracy.

- **Feel free to have more than one type of protein, vegetable or fruit at meals, as long as the total amount adds up to one serving.** For example, let's say for breakfast, which allows you to have one serving of fruit, you'd like to have blueberries and cherries. It's easy. Simply combine half a serving of blueberries with half a serving of cherries to make one serving.

- **Spice up your meals with herbs and spices.** Many herbs and spices have health-promoting properties in addition to enhancing flavors. Be sure to avoid using any spice mixes that contain sugar.

What does this look like on your plate? See the "Menu Days Menu Plan."

MENU DAYS MENU PLAN

BREAKFAST

1 Protein

1 Fruit OR 1 Grain

1 Beverage

MID-MORNING SNACK

1 Protein OR 1 Lean for Life protein snack

LUNCH

1 Protein

1 Vegetable

2 Cups greens

1 Salad dressing

1 Fruit

1 Beverage

MID-AFTERNOON SNACK

1 Protein OR 1 Lean for Life protein snack

DINNER

1 Protein

1 Vegetable

2 Cups greens

1 Salad dressing

1 Fruit

1 Beverage

EVENING SNACK

1 Protein OR 1 Lean for Life protein snack

WHAT TO DO EVERY SINGLE DAY DURING RAPID WEIGHT LOSS

Although you'll be following different menu plans on your Protein Days and Menu Days, you'll need to do the following *every day* whether it's a Protein Day or a Menu Day:

☐ **Drink at least 80 ounces of water or other calorie-free beverages per day.** Getting adequate hydration during the program is critical. Your thirst signals and hunger signals are controlled in the same region of the brain called the *hypothalamus*. This means that oftentimes when you *think* you're hungry, you may actually be just thirsty. Also, not getting enough fluids can pose a host of problems, including headaches, mental fuzziness and uncomfortable constipation. On this program, you may drink water or any calorie-free beverage to reach your target goal of 80 ounces per day. It is okay to drink caffeinated beverages, but be aware that consuming caffeine later in the day or in the evening may disrupt sleep, which—as you'll learn on Day 19 in chapter 6—can cause imbalances in your appetite hormones.

☐ **Take a sugar-free daily fiber supplement.** Fiber promotes a number of health benefits in addition to promoting bowel regularity.

☐ **You may add table salt to your food (unless you have high blood pressure).** This may help alleviate the slight dizziness some dieters occasionally experience.

☐ **Take vitamin and mineral supplements.** Vitamin and mineral supplements are an essential part of this program because they maximize absorption and utilization of the foods you eat, safeguard against nutritional deficiencies and enhance your weight-loss progress in a variety of ways. In addition to taking a high-quality multi-vitamin and mineral supplement during this program, our patients take a prescription-strength oral potassium chloride supplement to maintain healthy potassium levels. Potassium is also available over the counter in lower doses in the form of potassium gluconate. Table salt and salt substitutes also contain potassium. (*Important:* If you are being treated for chronic disease, have high blood pressure or are taking potassium-sparing diuretics, you should *not* take extra potassium supplements without first consulting your primary health-care provider.) Other supplements that can be beneficial—but are not mandatory—during weight loss include omega-3 fatty acids, gamma linolenic acid, capsinoids, B vitamins (especially B$_{12}$), vitamin D, magnesium, selenium and iron. You'll learn more about vitamins and minerals and how they can help on this program on Day 23 in chapter 7.

☐ **Take your ketostick reading every morning.** Using your ketostick, test for ketosis every morning. Here's how to do it to ensure an accurate reading. When you first get out of bed, empty your bladder and test your urine according to the instructions on the ketostick label. If your ketostick shows pink or purple, you are in ketosis. If you're not in ketosis, you may be eating too many carbohydrates. Keep in mind that going out of ketosis may initiate weight regain and may diminish the brain, body and gut benefits you have gained.

☐ **Record everything you eat and drink.** Becoming aware of what, when and why you eat is a critical part of this program. On Day 1 of Rapid Weight Loss (see page 64), you'll see how to track your daily intake.

☐ **Weigh yourself every morning.** Weigh yourself at the same time every morning, in the nude, after emptying your bladder.

☐ **Move more.** On this program, you're encouraged to "move more" by engaging in moderate physical activity on a daily basis, like walking. We recommend aiming for 10,000 steps a day, but it's important to build up to that gradually. Throughout the book, you'll learn much more about specific types of activities that can help shrink fat cells as well as enhance your mood and improve your health.

☐ **Stress less.** As you'll discover in upcoming chapters, chronic stress can stall your efforts to get lean. On the flip side, reducing stress can be beneficial to your progress. Use the techniques described in the book to help you "stress less."

☐ **Use mental training techniques.** Throughout the book, you'll find a variety of mental training strategies that, when used daily, will become powerful tools to help you become lean and healthy.

☐ **Choose a daily affirmation.** Choose a positive statement about yourself that you will repeat to yourself throughout the day. For information on how to create your affirmations, see Day 17 in chapter 6.

☐ **Use this book as a tool.** This book is designed to be your constant companion throughout the weight-loss process. After your first read, we urge you to re-read through it every day as you go through the program.

PHASE 3: METABOLIC ADJUSTMENT

Metabolic Adjustment is a critical two-week transition that draws on hormone science to allow you to eat more food *without gaining weight*. Guidelines for this phase are presented in chapter 8.

PHASE 4: METABOLIC EQUILIBRIUM

Metabolic Equilibrium is a lifestyle program to keep you Lean for Life. You'll discover the secrets to staying lean in chapter 9.

EAT BETTER
MOVE MORE
STRESS LESS

Practice the Lean for Life Mantra

At Lean for Life, our philosophy is simple. We do not expect you to strive for *perfection*. Instead, we urge you to try to do *better*.

EAT BETTER

You may not be able to eat *perfectly* every day, but you *can* "Eat Better." This program is designed to help you learn to make better food choices that will nourish your brain, body and gut—and satisfy your taste buds—in ways that help you get lean and stay lean.

MOVE MORE

You may not be able to dedicate a big chunk of time every day to exercise, but you can "Move More." This program will introduce you to easy ways to build more physical activity into your daily life.

STRESS LESS

You may not be able to eliminate stress from your life, but with the strategies presented here, you can learn to "Stress Less." During your program, you'll discover better ways to manage the stress that comes with everyday life.

LEAN FOODS

PROTEIN

On Protein Days, have a minimum of 6 protein servings. On Menu Days, have your choice of 1 protein serving each at breakfast, mid-morning snack, lunch, mid-afternoon snack, dinner and evening snack. Weigh meat, seafood and poultry (raw, skinned and boned) with all visible fat removed. Broil, boil, barbecue, microwave, roast, poach, bake or "fry" in a nonstick pan using a nonfat cooking spray.

FOOD CHOICE	SERVING SIZE	CARBOHYDRATES PER SERVING (GRAMS)
MEAT AND POULTRY SELECTIONS		
Beef flank	3½ ounces	0
Beef round	3½ ounces	0
Beef sirloin (ground, 7% fat maximum)	3 ounces	0
Bison	3½ ounces	0
Chicken breast (canned, white, water-packed)	2½ ounces	0
Chicken breast (fresh or frozen)	3½ ounces	0
Chicken breast (ground, 99% fat-free)	3½ ounces	0
Cold cuts (97-98% lean/fat-free)	2½ ounces	1
Pork tenderloin (lean)	3 ounces	0
Turkey (breast)	3½ ounces	0
Turkey breast (ground, 97% fat-free)	3½ ounces	0
Veal	3½ ounces	0
DAIRY SELECTIONS		
Almond milk (unsweetened)	1 cup	1
Cheese (fat-free or low-fat)	2 ounces	2
Cottage cheese (low-fat, plain)	4 ounces	4
Egg*	1	1

continued

LEAN FOODS

FOOD CHOICE	SERVING SIZE	CARBOHYDRATES PER SERVING (GRAMS)
Egg whites	2	1
Milk (nonfat)	1 cup	12
Soy milk	1 cup	10
Yogurt (Greek, nonfat)	1 cup	7
Yogurt (nonfat, plain)	1/2 cup	9
VEGETARIAN SELECTIONS		
Seitan	4 ounces	10
Tempeh	3 ounces	9
Tofu (low-fat)	6 ounces	2
Veggie burger	1/3 cup	3
Veggie cutlet	15 grams protein	<12
Other meat substitutes	15 grams protein	<12
SEAFOOD SELECTIONS		
Catfish	3 1/2 ounces	0
Cod	3 1/2 ounces	0
Crab	3 1/2 ounces	1
Haddock	3 1/2 ounces	0
Halibut**	3 1/2 ounces	0
Lobster	3 1/2 ounces	1
Orange Roughy	3 1/2 ounces	0
Perch	3 1/2 ounces	0
Salmon**	3 1/2 ounces	0
Scallops**	3 1/2 ounces	2
Sea bass	3 1/2 ounces	0

LEAN FOODS

FOOD CHOICE	SERVING SIZE	CARBOHYDRATES PER SERVING (GRAMS)
Shark	3½ ounces	0
Shrimp**	3½ ounces	1
Snapper**	3½ ounces	0
Sole	3½ ounces	0
Swordfish	3½ ounces	0
Trout (rainbow)	3½ ounces	0
Tuna** (white, fresh or frozen)	3½ ounces	0
Tuna** (canned or packaged white albacore, water-packed)	2½ ounces	0
Turbot	3½ ounces	0
White fish	3½ ounces	0

LEAN FOR LIFE PROTEIN PRODUCTS***

   * Look for eggs that are DHA-enriched for a good source of omega-3 fatty acids.
   ** High in omega-3 fatty acids.
   *** Lean for Life products count as 1 protein serving.

SMART CARBS: GRAINS

On Menu Days, your breakfast includes your choice of either 1 serving of fruit OR 1 serving of grain from the following list. When shopping for cereals, pay close attention to nutrition labels and look for brands with fewer than 100 calories per serving and up to 20 grams of carbohydrates per serving.

Bread (whole grain, up to 80 calories)	1 slice	<15
Cream of Rice	½ cup	14
Cream of Wheat	½ cup	13
Oatmeal (cooked)	½ cup	12
Quinoa (cooked)	⅓ cup	13

continued

LEAN FOODS

FOOD CHOICE	SERVING SIZE	CARBOHYDRATES PER SERVING (GRAMS)
Shredded Wheat	¾ cup	23
Whole-wheat tortillas (low carb)	6" diameter	12

SMART CARBS: VEGETABLES

On Menu Days, your choice of 1 serving at lunch and at dinner. Measure raw, frozen (thawed) or water packed (drained), unless otherwise stated. No sugar added. Have 2 cups torn lettuce at lunch and dinner.

Food	Serving	Carbs
Asparagus	1 cup	8
Bean sprouts	1 cup	14
Broccoli	1 cup	5
Cabbage	1 cup	4
Carrots	½ cup	8
Cauliflower	1 cup	5
Celery	1 cup	6
Chinese pea pods	1 cup	11
Collard greens	1 cup	8
Cucumbers	1 cup	3
Jicama	½ cup	5
Kale	1 cup	7
Lettuce	2 cups	3
Mushrooms (raw)	2 cups	7
Mustard greens	1 cup	3
Okra	1 cup	8
Onion	½ cup	6
Pepper (red, green, orange, yellow)	1 small	4
Sauerkraut	1 cup	10

LEAN FOODS

FOOD CHOICE	SERVING SIZE	CARBOHYDRATES PER SERVING (GRAMS)
Spinach (cooked)	1 cup	7
Spinach (raw)	2 cups	4
String beans	1 cup	8
Tomato	1 small	5
Zucchini	1 cup	4

SMART CARBS: FRUITS

On Menu Days, your choice of 1 serving at breakfast (when not choosing a grain), lunch and dinner. Include at least one citrus fruit per day. Choose fresh, frozen (thawed) or water packed (without sugar or fruit juice).

Apple	1 small (2" diameter)	17
Applesauce (unsweetened)	½ cup	14
Apricots (fresh)	2 medium	9
Banana	½ small	13
Blackberries	⅔ cup	12
Blueberries	⅔ cup	14
Boysenberries	⅔ cup	11
Cantaloupe	¾ cup	11
Casaba melon	½ cup	6
Cherries	10	11
Dates	2	13
Grapefruit*	½ cup	9
Honeydew melon	½ cup	7
Kiwi	1 medium (3 ounces)	11

continued

LEAN FOODS

FOOD CHOICE	SERVING SIZE	CARBOHYDRATES PER SERVING (GRAMS)
Mango (sliced)	1/2 cup	14
Nectarine (sliced)	1/2 cup	8
Orange*	1 small (2 1/2" diameter)	14
Papaya (cubed)	1/2 cup	7
Peach	1 small (2 1/2" diameter)	10
Pear (Bartlett)	1/2 small or 2 1/2 ounces	13
Persimmon	1	8
Pineapple (cubed)	1/2 cup	10
Raisins	1/2 ounce	11
Raspberries	2/3 cup	10
Rhubarb	1 cup	7
Strawberries	1 cup	11
Tangerine*	1 (2 1/2" diameter)	9
Watermelon (cubed)	1/2 cup	6

*Citrus fruit

MISCELLANEOUS

Your choice of 1 serving, twice per day, with the meals of your choice.

Coffee creamer (nondairy, powdered, fat-free)	1 teaspoon	2
Gelatin (diet)	1/2 cup	0
Green onion (tops)	1 teaspoon	0
Horseradish	1 teaspoon	1
Margarine (nonfat, 5 calories maximum)	1 tablespoon	0

LEAN FOODS

FOOD CHOICE	SERVING SIZE	CARBOHYDRATES PER SERVING (GRAMS)
Mustard	1 teaspoon	0
Peppers, jalapeno	2 small	2
Pimento	2 small	1
Radishes	2 medium	1
Vinegar (unseasoned)	2 tablespoons	2

BEVERAGES

Water

Coffee*

Decaffeinated coffee

Tea (hot or iced, unsweetened or with sugar-free substitute)*

Herbal tea

Diet soda*

Diet seltzer water

Diet mineral water

Any other calorie-free drink

*This beverage may contain caffeine, which may stimulate appetite or make you feel jumpy or "wired." If you choose drinks containing caffeine, you may want to limit them. If you reduce or eliminate caffeine, do it gradually to prevent withdrawal symptoms that often occur when stopping "cold turkey."

SALAD DRESSINGS

Any fat-free dressing, up to 15 calories and 3 grams carbohydrates OR 1 teaspoon olive, canola, walnut or flaxseed oil

Lettuce	2 cups

Remember you can find more extensive, detailed food lists on our website (leanforlife.com).

View more detailed food lists.

THEN & WOW!

42
POUNDS LOST!

Rob Douglis

AGE
44

OCCUPATION
Investment Consultant

HEIGHT
6'0"

CURRENT WEIGHT
192

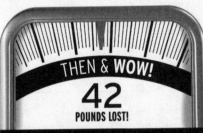

WAIST MANAGEMENT
I'm down from a 42-inch waist to a 35.

There's nothing more humbling than glancing at a group work photo, wondering 'who's that big guy?' and realizing it's you! Thanks to the Lean for Life program, I've maintained a 42-pound weight loss for nearly four years. These days, when I look at a photo of myself, I actually like the guy I see.

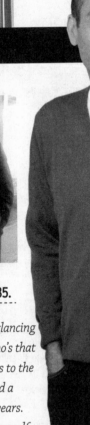

PHOTOS DON'T LIE: I attended a work party, and someone was taking group photos. When I later saw the pictures, I was embarrassed to see how large my stomach was. That's when I knew it was time to make a change. Two women I was working with had done very well on the Lean for Life program, so I trusted it would work for me.

MINDFUL EATING: I used to eat whenever I was stressed or bored. These days, I work out instead. I'm also much more conscious and deliberate about what I eat—and how much. I can't remember the last time I ate rice, bread, pasta or any kind of salad dressing. It's not that I can't have those foods—I just no longer want them.

DENYING DENIAL: Before I lost weight, I ate what I wanted, when I wanted it. The program not only taught me how and what to eat for optimal health, but it also provided the structure I really needed. I think most of us underestimate how much we eat and overestimate how active we are. When you're completing a Daily Action Plan every day, there's no mystery. It kept me honest about what and how much I was eating, as well as how active I was.

HEALTHY ROLE MODEL: One thing I love about becoming healthier is that I'm showing my teenage kids that you can achieve anything when you set a goal, stay focused and motivated, and fully commit to accomplishing it.

BIG CHANGES: When I was overweight, I was unhappy and embarrassed. Now, my energy—and my self-confidence—are at all-time highs. I've been in a great relationship with my girlfriend for three years now, and my overall outlook on life is just so much more positive. It know it sounds like a cliché to say I feel like a new man, but I really do!

3 THE THREE-DAY PREP TO PRIME YOUR BRAIN, BODY AND GUT FOR SUCCESS

You may be feeling so eager to jump right into Rapid Weight Loss that you may be tempted to skip over this chapter. Don't! Before you dive into Rapid Weight Loss, it's very important to prepare your brain, body and gut for success. We have developed a three-day crash course to help you do just that. What we've developed may seem counterintuitive, but years of practical experience with many thousands of patients have shown us that those who follow the Prep tend to feel better and achieve greater results during Rapid Weight Loss.

In this chapter, you'll discover why the Prep is so beneficial to your weight-loss success. Plus, you'll get a day-by-day guide for doing your own Prep at home, including detailed instructions on what to eat. Surprise! Eating high-fat fare like pizza or cheeseburgers is okay during the Prep!

BENEFITS OF DOING THE PREP

- **Transition comfortably into Rapid Weight Loss.** Starting a new program can be a real shock to the system, both physically and mentally. The Prep eases you into the structured four-week program.
- **Satisfy any lingering cravings.** This is your chance to indulge—but not overindulge—in some of the high-fat foods you crave before you begin Rapid Weight Loss.

- **Replenish your body's reserves of essential fatty acids and amino acids.** If you've already been following a low-fat diet or restricting calories for two weeks or more prior to this, your levels of essential fatty acids and amino acids may be depleted. Replenishing your reserves helps maintain gallbladder health.

- **Prepare yourself mentally.** During the Prep, you'll begin the process of training your brain to help you lose weight.

- **Zero in on powerful motivators that will help you stay on track throughout your program.** Knowing *why* you want to become Lean for Life is essential to your success. Our clinic nurses tell us that the patients who are more in touch with what is motivating them to lose weight tend to have better results.

- **Set goals that increase your chances for success.** Setting goals that are too lofty, too vague or too low can put you on the fast track to failure. The Prep shows you how to set goals that will motivate you: goals that you can—and will—achieve.

- **Stock up on all the tools and foods you'll need.** This is the time for you to make a quick trip to the grocery store, clear some of the junk food out of your kitchen and gather all the materials you'll need (don't worry, there aren't many) for the four-week program.

- **Protect your gallbladder.** Being overweight or obese increases your risk for gallbladder disease, and losing weight rapidly through dieting may exacerbate an existing gallbladder condition. A dramatic reduction in dietary fat can contribute to the problem. The foods you'll be eating during the Prep will supply the fat your body needs to reduce this risk. Rest assured that throughout the Rapid Weight Loss phase, you'll also be eating foods that contain reduced, but adequate, amounts of fat to minimize the risk of gallbladder problems. (If you have a history of gallbladder disease or any symptoms associated with it—such as attacks of sharp pain in your upper-right abdomen, usually accompanied by nausea or gas and bloating after eating—check with your doctor before beginning any diet program.)

THE PREP RULES

The guidelines for the three-day Prep are simple and straightforward. As you'll see, during this phase, you are allowed to indulge in some of your favorite foods, but that doesn't mean the Prep is a "last hurrah" during which you can pig out uncontrollably. People who make this mistake can gain as much as 10 pounds in just three days. Why set the starting line back when you don't need to?

- **Eat three complete meals a day.** Meals should include a protein food, a salad with dressing, a potato or other starch, vegetables, fresh fruit, and milk or the calorie-free beverage of your choice. See the "Sample Prep Day Menu."

- **Include the high-fat foods you crave at mealtimes.** If there are certain high-fat foods you crave—pizza, cheeseburgers, lasagna—you may have them now as part of your meals. This is an opportunity to satisfy any nagging cravings you have before you begin Rapid Weight Loss.

- **Eat protein-based snacks between meals.** Good options include a slice of deli turkey wrapped around cheese, a handful of nuts or seeds, celery with peanut butter, or Greek yogurt.

- **Avoid or limit desserts and alcohol.** Remember, the Prep is not a free-for-all. Do your best to say no to candy, cookies, cakes, and pies, as well as margaritas, Mai Tais, and Manhattan Sours. Sugar-laden foods, refined carbohydrates and alcohol can trigger cravings and stimulate your appetite.

- **Start taking your vitamins and supplements.** See the recommendations in chapter 2 (page 34).

- **Drink at least 80 ounces of calorie-free fluids a day.** Water is the best option, but you can drink any calorie-free beverage you prefer.

- **Don't make any big changes to your physical activity habits yet.** If you currently follow any sort of workout routine, continue doing so. If you don't exercise, try taking a 10-minute walk.

- **Begin taking a sugar-free daily fiber supplement.** See the recommendations in chapter 2 (page 34).

SAMPLE PREP DAY MENU

BREAKFAST

2 eggs or omelette

Bacon, ham or sausage (if desired)

1 slice whole-wheat toast with butter

6-8 ounces unsweetened orange juice

LUNCH

Tuna salad sandwich or pizza

Green salad with dressing

Vegetable

Fresh fruit

Coffee or any calorie-free beverage

DINNER

6 ounces steak or fish

Baked potato with butter and sour cream

Green salad with dressing

Vegetable

Fruit or other dessert

Coffee or any calorie-free beverage

SNACKS

Cheese, nuts, seeds, celery with peanut butter, yogurt

The Inside Story from Dr. Allouche

PEPTIDE POWER

Do you ever feel hungry even after you've just eaten a big meal? Eating more protein, as you'll be doing on this program, can help you keep hunger at bay. The scientific community has long known that protein helps suppress people's appetites, but we are just now beginning to understand why. Research in a 2012 issue of the journal *Cell* points to peptides, which are molecules found in the protein you consume. These peptides set in motion a series of signals that fend off hunger. Here's how they do it.

Imagine that the peptides have cell phones. Once the protein arrives in your intestines, the peptides start sending out a flurry of text messages: *Feeling full, no need to eat for a while.*☺ Tiny receivers called *mu-opioid receptors* nearby intercept the messages and forward them to your nervous system, which in turn forwards them to your brain. Your brain responds directly to your gut with a text saying: *Increase glucose synthesis ASAP.* Glucose synthesis, also known as *neoglucogenesis,* is an internal process that relays another message to the liver, which forwards it to the areas of the brain that control food intake, telling them to *suppress appetite.*

The result? You've heard of a vicious cycle—well, this is the exact opposite. It's like the peptides have created a dieter's "BFF (best friends forever) cycle" in which a continuous loop of hunger-reducing messages between your gut, brain and nervous system help keep you feeling fuller for longer. And all you have to do to take advantage of the BFF cycle is eat your protein as recommended on this program.

THE PREP: DAY 1

EASY DOES IT

It's Prep Day 1, and you may be wondering if this part of the program is really necessary. It is! Even though this day is not designed to activate weight loss, it is very important to the weight-loss process because it requires you to engage in some of the key habits that are at the foundation of the Lean for Life program. Specifically, you'll begin using food to modify your biochemistry, you'll begin harnessing your brainpower to work for you instead of against you and you'll begin taking an active role to make this plan work for you.

INGREDIENTS FOR SUCCESS

Today is a great day to gather up the supplies you'll need for this program. You can find most items in your local drugstore, from online retailers or on our website (leanforlife.com).

- Ketone strips (known as Fat-Burning Indicators to us Lean for Lifers).
- Food scale.
- Measuring cups and spoons.
- Water bottle (30 ounces or larger).
- Tape measure.
- Pedometer, accelerometer or other physical activity monitoring device.
- Weight scale.
- High PER protein snacks.

WHAT'S YOUR MOTIVATION?

To get the most out of your efforts, it's important to understand what's motivating you to become Lean for Life. What was the "final straw" that pushed you to start this program? For Andrea, it was a clothes shopping trip that ended in tears and embarrassment when the sales clerk took one look at her and said, "Oh, honey, we don't have anything here that would fit you. You should try that plus-size shop down the street." For Brad, it was when his brother Gabe posted a vacation photo of the two of them wearing swimming trunks on a social media site, and the comments were less than kind. For 32-year-old Kendall, it was when her doctor told her she was pre-diabetic, had high cholesterol and high blood pressure, and if she didn't lose weight, she would have to go on medication for the rest of her life. And for Julia, it was the mortifying moment when that cute coworker she'd been eyeing for a while finally came up to talk to her and asked her when her baby was due—even though she wasn't pregnant.

What was *your* final straw?

Your final straw may have been the thing that pushed you over the edge to do something about your weight, but it isn't necessarily the thing that will keep you motivated throughout the program. You also need to understand the underlying reasons—negative and positive—that are driving you to become Lean for Life. What's driving you?

Think of all the things associated with being overweight that affect your life negatively. How has the extra weight impacted your health, relationships, social life, career and self-confidence? Jot down a couple—just a few, don't go overboard here—of negative aspects of being overweight that you will not miss when you become Lean for Life. Here are a few that we hear often:

I'm embarrassed to go shopping for clothes.

I hate the way I look.

I feel tired all the time.

When you think about these things, how does it make you feel? Pretty lousy, huh?

Now, switch your thinking to the benefits you'll enjoy after achieving your ideal lean weight. Sit down with a stack of 3 x 5 note cards or small pieces of paper, and on each one, write down one positive thing you'll like. Now's the time to go overboard and include all the good things that come to mind.

Clothes shopping will be fun.

I'll be a better role model for my kids.

I'll have lots of energy to do the things I want to do in life.

I'll look great at my reunion.

I'll feel more in control.

I'll be healthier so I will be around longer to see my kids grow up.

I'll feel more confident about myself in the dating world.

I'll want to make love with the lights on again.

How do you feel now after writing down all these positive benefits? A lot better than before, right? Before we complete this exercise, we want to let you in on a little secret—you've just done your first mental training session. We'll go into this in much more detail later, but by simply focusing your thoughts on the negatives and then willfully shifting your thoughts to the positives, you're setting in motion changes in your brain and biochemistry that will help you lose weight. Pretty cool, isn't it?

Now, back to the exercise. After you've written down all your reasons, prioritize them. Move the cards around until you've clarified your top five reasons for becoming Lean for Life.

Now write down your top five on three note cards or pieces of paper to create a powerful tool we call "My Motivator Cards." Keep one in your purse or wallet. Put the second where you're sure to see it every morning—in your medicine chest, on your bathroom mirror or in your underwear drawer. Keep the third in a desk drawer at the office, in your gym bag, in your glove compartment or in your Daily Action Plan (DAP—see page 64). In today's digital world, it's also a good idea to keep a copy of your top five on your computer, on your smart phone and on your tablet, too.

Review your "My Motivator Cards" daily and whenever temptation presents itself. Whenever you feel like swinging by the bakery on your way to work or ordering a piece of cheesecake for dessert, for example, take a look at your list. These reminders will help keep you focused on why you're investing the time and energy to lose weight.

TODAY'S ACTION CHECKLIST

- Follow the Prep Rules (page 48).
- Get supplies.
- Create your "My Motivator Cards."

THE PREP: DAY 2

START AT THE FINISH LINE: SETTING GOALS

One of your tasks today is to zero in on your long-term ideal lean weight—not what you want to weigh a week from now, but what you'd like to weigh when you're Lean for Life. Is your goal to fit into the skinny jeans you used to wear in college, to fit into the size 10 wedding dress you bought for your upcoming nuptials or to lower your Body Mass Index (BMI) from "obese" to "healthy"? Only you can determine what your "ideal lean weight" is. When you're coming up with your goal, keep in mind these common-sense guidelines:

- **Be realistic.** Saying you want to lose 30 pounds in one week or drop 10 inches from your waistline in three weeks is unrealistic and sets you up for failure. Choose a goal that is attainable. On this program, you can lose up to 20 pounds in 28 days.

- **Make it measurable.** There's an old adage that says, "If you can't measure it, you can't manage it." That definitely applies to weight loss. You need to be able to measure your success. See the "Motivating Measurements" in the section that follows.

When you have determined your ideal lean weight goal, write it down in the "Starting Measurements" form in Appendix E. The simple act of writing it down makes it more "real" and makes you feel more accountable, which makes you more likely to achieve it.

MOTIVATING MEASUREMENTS

Here are a number of simple ways to measure your progress that can help keep you motivated.

- **Weigh yourself.** Weighing yourself, which you'll be doing every morning from now on, is the most obvious way to measure your progress, but it isn't the only one.

- **Measure up.** Using a tape measure, measure your waist, chest, lower abdomen, hips, and upper-thigh area, and record the numbers in the "Weekly Progress Report" form in Appendix F. You'll be asked to take these same measurements once a week, which is a very effective way to monitor fat loss.

- **Know your BMI.** Refer to the "Body Mass Index (BMI) Chart" in Appendix D to find your BMI.

- **Calculate your waist-to-height ratio.** Waist-to-height ratio is a way to measure body fat distribution. It's also a very simple way to determine if your size is putting you at an increased risk for serious health complications like type 2 diabetes, high blood pressure and heart disease. It couldn't be simpler to calculate. Basically, keeping your waist circumference to less than half your height reduces your risk. For example, if you're 5'4" (64 inches), your waist should measure less than 32 inches. If you're 6' tall (72 inches), it's best to keep your waist under 36 inches. To measure your waist accurately, hold the measuring tape about 1 inch above your belly button.

- **Let your clothing give you clues.** Do you have a favorite pair of jeans, trousers, or a shirt or dress that is feeling a little tighter than it used to? Place the item in the back of your closet and write yourself a reminder to try it on again two weeks from now. Still too tight? Try again two weeks later. You'll know you're making progress when the item feels comfortable or even a bit loose. The way your clothes fit can be a great way to gauge your progress.

WHERE ARE YOU TODAY?

In order to measure your progress throughout your weight-loss journey, you need to know where you stand today. Take and record your "Starting Measurements" today and record them in Appendix E (page 251).

MEASURE YOUR FEELINGS, TOO

Based on our experience with so many people who have gone through this program, we have found that in addition to tracking the changes in your physical body, it's a good idea to take note of changes that are happening on the inside, too. We're talking about the way you feel. Take the "Quiz: What's Your PSQ (Personal Satisfaction Quotient)?" to see where you stand.

QUIZ: WHAT'S YOUR PSQ
(PERSONAL SATISFACTION QUOTIENT)?

How you feel about your life—your work, your family, your relationships, your finances, your health, your body—impacts everything you think, say and do. Are you physically energetic? Are you happy more often than sad? Do you get along with others? Do you like yourself? Circle the number that reflects how you feel about your life at this moment:

1	2	3	4	5	6	7	8	9	10

I've never been
more unhappy

I'm generally satisfied
with my life

My life is
terrific!

TODAY'S ACTION CHECKLIST

- ■ Follow the Prep Rules (page 48).
- ■ Determine your ideal lean weight.
- ■ Weigh yourself.
- ■ Take and record your measurements.
- ■ Find your BMI.
- ■ Calculate your waist-to-height ratio.
- ■ Put "too-tight" clothes away and try them on two weeks from now.

THE PREP: DAY 3

MASTER THE BRAIN-BODY-GUT CONNECTION

Embarrassment makes you blush. Feeling nervous makes your skin itch. Watching an awe-inspiring performance by your favorite musical artist gives you goose bumps. Recalling a frightening event makes your hands cold and clammy. Reading a text from that special someone gets your heart racing. These are all examples of the "mind-body connection," a concept that's become so commonplace over the past decade that a simple internet search for that term brings up nearly 50 million results. In fact, that's how we first described it over 15 years ago, but we've now learned that it's really a "brain-body-gut connection."

New science has revealed that the connection between your brain, body chemistry and gut health is undeniable. Your brain is responsible for the thoughts you think, the emotions you feel and the images you see, all of which affect your body chemistry. Likewise, your body chemistry has an effect on your brain and subsequently, all your thoughts, feelings and impressions. Your gut also plays an important role in your thoughts and feelings, releasing neurotransmitters involved in regulating moods and emotions. All of this impacts your behavior, which in turn affects your brain, body chemistry and gut health. It's an endless loop that is either working to keep you fat or helping you get and stay lean.

Every part of this program is designed to help you get out of that vicious circle and into a more health-promoting loop that encourages weight loss. Our goal is to give you the tools that will outsmart your biology and make the brain-body-gut connection work positively for you. If you're feeling sorry for yourself, we'll encourage you to do things that will give you pleasure. If just thinking about exercise makes you tired, we'll help you learn to think about it differently. If you're feeling edgy, we'll offer ways to relax. If you're frustrated, we'll share success stories of others who've experienced the same feelings and overcome them. If you're overwhelmed, we'll suggest ways to refocus your thoughts and energy.

Together we'll explore the importance of treating yourself well and cultivating an "achievement attitude." You'll learn how to plan ahead for each day's obstacles, how to mentally rehearse situations to enhance your success, and how to change your brain and body chemistry through your habits and behaviors. One of the things our patients find most surprising and most exciting about this program is that it is possible to learn successful weight-loss strategies. You don't have to be born lean; you can *learn to become lean.* And your brain, body and gut can help you do it. Today, you're going to start putting this concept to work with a simple visualization exercise.

VISUALIZE YOUR SUCCESS

No matter how enthusiastic you are when you start your program, it's easy to lose momentum after the initial excitement fades. That's why it's vital to have a visual reminder of your goals. Here are a few ideas that have helped other Lean for Lifers stay on course. Choose whichever appeals to you most, or come up with your own motivational idea. Whatever you do, make sure it's a graphic reminder of why you're doing this program.

- **Find an "After" photo of yourself.** You may have to dig through boxes or photo albums, or scroll through your online photo library, but find a picture of yourself when you were leaner and healthier. Choose one that captures the physical image you want to project again.

- **Find a role model "After" photo.** If you don't have any real photos available, thumb through magazines or download images of people who look the way you would like to look. Be sure to focus on overall body image rather than facial features or hairstyles. And whatever you do, be practical. Don't set yourself up for failure by choosing images that are completely unrealistic. Nothing can be more demoralizing than comparing yourself to an airbrushed actor or model. You may find it helpful to do this exercise with someone you trust who can give you honest feedback as to what body type is realistic and appropriate.

- **Create an "After" photo of yourself.** Alice, who succeeded on this program, came up with a clever way to visualize her leaner body. She asked her daughter to take several pictures of her wearing a one-piece bathing suit. She selected one of the pictures as her "Before" photo and used a second one from the same session to create her "After" shot. Alice took a fine-line pen and outlined her leaner, healthier body shape on the photo. Using a pair of manicure scissors, she trimmed away the weight she was determined to lose. With a few snips, she had created an image that motivated her to pursue her goal.

- **Use web tools to create an "After" photo.** You don't have to be crafty like Alice to visualize what you would look like leaner. Several websites, such as weightview.com, will do all the "leanifying" for you. Just submit a photo, tell them how much weight you want to lose, and they'll digitally alter your image to show you what you would look like leaner.

It's your future. Picture it now!

WATCH YOUR PROGRESS BEFORE YOUR EYES

If you want to see your progress as it occurs, today is the day to plan for it. Take a "Before" photo today that you can use to compare to future photos so you can visually track your progress as you lose weight. Here are a few tips for taking good "Before" and "After" pictures.

- Take photos in a well-lit space.
- Wear clothing that shows your shape rather than hiding it.
- Ask a friend to take the photos or use a tripod.
- Take photos at the same time of day so the lighting is similar.
- Stand the same distance from the camera each time.
- Take a variety of poses—facing the camera, at a 45-degree angle, sideways and back-facing the camera.

You can also take advantage of a number of fun web tools and apps that can help you see your progress as it unfolds. One app (watchmechangeapp.com) has you upload a daily photo and then after you reach your goal, it will create a short video of your weight-loss progression.

For additional encouragement, check out the many "Before" and "After" photos on our website (leanforlife.com) and feel free to share your own success story after you complete the program (lindora.com/share-success-story.aspx).

LET'S GO SHOPPING!

Today is the ideal time to hit the grocery store to stock up on the foods you'll be eating on the program. You'll find a handy "Lean for Life Shopping List" following the Action Checklist for Day 3, or you can download one from our website (leanforlife.com). Just check off the items you want to buy that day, take it with you to the store, and stick to it!

Access the Lean for Life Shopping List.

TODAY'S ACTION CHECKLIST

- ■ Follow the Prep Rules (page 48).
- ■ Create an "After" photo.
- ■ Take a "Before" photo.
- ■ Use the Lean for Life Shopping List and go grocery shopping.

LEAN FOR LIFE SHOPPING LIST

MEAT AND POULTRY

- ☐ Beef flank
- ☐ Beef round
- ☐ Beef sirloin (ground, 7% fat maximum)
- ☐ Chicken breast (canned, water-packed)
- ☐ Chicken breast (fresh or frozen)
- ☐ Chicken (ground white meat)
- ☐ Cold cuts (97-98% fat-free)
- ☐ Pork tenderloin (lean)
- ☐ Turkey (breast, 97% fat-free)
- ☐ Turkey (ground, 97% fat-free)
- ☐ Veal

continued

SEAFOOD

- [ ] Catfish
- [ ] Cod
- [ ] Crab
- [ ] Haddock
- [ ] Halibut
- [ ] Lobster
- [ ] Orange roughy
- [ ] Perch
- [ ] Salmon
- [ ] Scallops
- [ ] Sea bass
- [ ] Shark
- [ ] Shrimp
- [ ] Snapper
- [ ] Sole
- [ ] Swordfish
- [ ] Trout (rainbow)
- [ ] Tuna (fresh or frozen)
- [ ] Tuna (white albacore, water-packed)
- [ ] Turbot
- [ ] White fish

PRODUCE

- [ ] Apples (small 2 ½" diameter)
- [ ] Applesauce (unsweetened)
- [ ] Apricots
- [ ] Asparagus
- [ ] Bananas (small)
- [ ] Blackberries
- [ ] Blueberries
- [ ] Boysenberries
- [ ] Broccoli
- [ ] Cabbage
- [ ] Cantaloupe
- [ ] Carrots
- [ ] Casaba melon
- [ ] Cauliflower
- [ ] Celery
- [ ] Cherries
- [ ] Chinese pea pods
- [ ] Cucumbers
- [ ] Dates
- [ ] Grapefruit
- [ ] Green beans
- [ ] Green onion (tops)
- [ ] Honeydew
- [ ] Jicama
- [ ] Kale
- [ ] Kiwi
- [ ] Lemons
- [ ] Lettuce
- [ ] Limes
- [ ] Mangoes
- [ ] Mushrooms
- [ ] Nectarines
- [ ] Okra
- [ ] Onions
- [ ] Oranges (small)
- [ ] Papaya
- [ ] Peaches (small)
- [ ] Pears (Bartlett)
- [ ] Peppers (yellow, green, red, orange)
- [ ] Peppers (jalapeño)
- [ ] Persimmons
- [ ] Pineapple
- [ ] Radishes
- [ ] Raisins
- [ ] Raspberries
- [ ] Rhubarb
- [ ] Sauerkraut
- [ ] Spinach
- [ ] Strawberries
- [ ] Tangerines
- [ ] Tomatoes
- [ ] Watermelon
- [ ] Zucchini

REFRIGERATED SECTION

- ☐ Cheese (fat-free, low-fat)
- ☐ Cottage cheese (low-fat, plain)
- ☐ Eggs (DHA enriched)
- ☐ Egg substitute
- ☐ Egg whites
- ☐ Margarine (nonfat)
- ☐ Tofu (low-fat)
- ☐ Veggie burger
- ☐ Veggie cutlet
- ☐ Yogurt (Greek, nonfat)
- ☐ Yogurt (nonfat, plain)

BEVERAGES

- ☐ Coffee
- ☐ Diet mineral water
- ☐ Diet seltzer
- ☐ Diet soda
- ☐ Milk (nonfat)
- ☐ Tea (black, green, herbal)
- ☐ Water
- ☐ Any other calorie-free beverage

GRAINS

- ☐ Cereal (less than 20 carbs)
- ☐ Cream of Rice
- ☐ Cream of Wheat
- ☐ Malt-O-Meal
- ☐ Oatmeal
- ☐ Whole-grain bread (less than 80 calories, less than 15 carbs)

SALAD OILS, DRESSINGS AND COOKING SPRAY

- ☐ Canola oil
- ☐ Canola oil spray
- ☐ Flaxseed oil
- ☐ Olive oil
- ☐ Olive oil spray
- ☐ Safflower spray
- ☐ Salad dressing (fat-free, up to 15 calories, up to 3 grams of carbs)
- ☐ Vinegar

FROZEN FOODS

- ☐ Chicken breast
- ☐ Fruits (see "Produce," no sugar added)
- ☐ Seafood (see "Seafood")
- ☐ Turkey burgers
- ☐ Veggie burgers
- ☐ Vegetables (see "Produce," no creams or sauces)

MISCELLANEOUS

- ☐ Creamer (powdered)
- ☐ Gelatin (diet)
- ☐ Horseradish
- ☐ Mustard
- ☐ Pimento

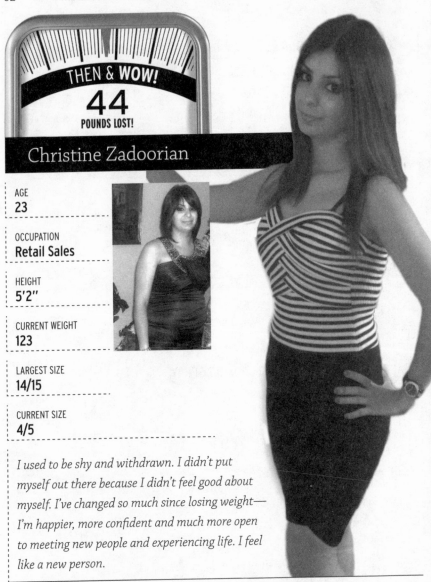

THEN & WOW!

44
POUNDS LOST!

Christine Zadoorian

AGE
23

OCCUPATION
Retail Sales

HEIGHT
5'2"

CURRENT WEIGHT
123

LARGEST SIZE
14/15

CURRENT SIZE
4/5

I used to be shy and withdrawn. I didn't put myself out there because I didn't feel good about myself. I've changed so much since losing weight—I'm happier, more confident and much more open to meeting new people and experiencing life. I feel like a new person.

THE COMPARISON TRAP: I grew up as the fat girl in a family of thin people. My parents, my brother and both my sisters have always been on the thin side. And then there was me. It was never fun or easy being compared to my sisters, but people did it all the time. I often felt judged and unattractive. A guy I worked with once asked me why I was so fat when my sister was thin. He speculated that I "sure must eat a lot." People can be incredibly brutal and insensitive.

DOCTOR'S ORDERS: When I complained to my doctor about how much my knees hurt, he told me I was overweight and that losing 40 pounds would make a world of difference. I was a little insulted, but I knew in my heart he was right. When you're carrying an extra 40 pounds, you don't realize how much added pressure it puts on your back, legs, knees and feet.

SUCCESS, AND THEN SOME: When I started the Lean for Life program, my original goal was to lose 30 pounds. But once I started losing and got into the groove, I allowed myself to dream bigger and to be honest about what I really, truly wanted for myself. I ended up exceeding my goal by nearly 50 percent.

KEEP MOVING: I work as a sales associate for a major department store, so I'm always on my feet. Before I lost weight, I often had knee pain from standing so long. I didn't move any more than I had to. But after I began the Lean for Life program, I made a conscious effort to start moving more at work. These days, I'm never in one place too long. A lot of people think being active means running or biking for an hour, but it can also mean just walking at work, taking the stairs instead of the elevator or parking in the first spot you see rather than circling for a closer space. A little movement here, a little movement there. Over time, it adds up to more calories burned and more pounds lost.

FULL CIRCLE: Not long ago, I ran into the guy who asked me why I was so fat and my sister was thin. As I was walking by, he called out my sister's name. He mistook me for the sister he once compared me to! While I lost the weight for myself, I have to admit the look on his face when he realized his mistake was icing on the cake—and a great reminder of just how far I've come.

4 RAPID WEIGHT LOSS WEEK 1:
CURB CRAVINGS AND START DROPPING POUNDS

If you've ever been on a diet, you know that the first few days tend to be the toughest. That's because this is the period when your brain, body and gut are still locked in the conspiracy mode you learned about in chapter 2. In these early days, the "BBG gang" fights back most vigorously against the changes you're making. Rest assured, we can help you through it. Going day by day, this chapter spells out simple strategies for succeeding in the critical first week. The tips and directions in this chapter have been collected from more than 15 million visits with patients and are meant to zero in on what you may be thinking, feeling and physically experiencing on each specific day of the program.

DAY 1: PROTEIN DAY

LET YOUR DAILY ACTION PLAN BE YOUR GUIDE

On Day 1, it's normal to feel excited but also a bit overwhelmed, which explains why the most common thing our nurses hear when patients start the program is: "Just tell me what I'm supposed to do." You may be thinking the same thing. To guide you through the first day—and every day thereafter on the program— we've created a Daily Action Plan (DAP).

EAT BETTER
MOVE MORE
STRESS LESS

Today is the first of your three initial Protein Days. Follow the step-by-step guidelines in chapter 2 (pages 27–30). Aim for one protein serving approximately every two hours. If you feel hungry, eat more frequently. To achieve ketosis, select protein servings that are low in carbohydrates.

One of the most powerful tools to becoming Lean for Life, the DAP is a simple daily record that will be your constant companion as you learn to eat better, move more and stress less. It is critical to your success. Just ask some of our patients, who have all found different reasons why it is essential to "Do the DAP."

- **Jodi, who lost 42 pounds,** likes to think of her DAP as a cheerleader that encourages her to develop healthy new habits.

- **Sarah, who dropped 18 pounds,** loves that her DAP helps her plan ways to overcome daily obstacles.

- **Janine, who is back in her "skinny jeans"** for the first time since giving birth to twins eight years ago, finds that spending just a few minutes a day filling out her DAP provides valuable feedback that makes her aware of what's working and areas where she may need a little help.

- **Joseph, who went from a pants size 38 to a 34,** is grateful that his DAP acts as a sort of friendly cop that keeps him accountable for his actions.

It won't take long for you to discover how doing the DAP helps you become your best self. If you're wondering why it's a "daily" action plan rather than a weekly or monthly plan, it's because losing weight by making changes to your habits and behaviors happens one day at a time. You need to plan on a daily basis, and you need to take *action* on a daily basis in order to create the new habits that will help you achieve a new look.

To make this easier, we've created helpful DAP sheets that are geared specifically to either Protein Days or Menu Days. In Appendix A, you'll find a completed "DAP for Menu Days–Sample," as well as blank sheets for "DAP for Protein Days" and "DAP for Menu Days." You'll also find blank sheets for DAPs for every phase of the program. You can either make copies of these or purchase our DAP booklet through our website (leanforlife.com). Or if you're enrolled in our online program, you can fill out your DAP online.

Fortunately, it takes only a few brief moments throughout the day to "Do the DAP." Here are step-by-step instructions.

FILL OUT THE WEEK, DAY AND DATE

Fill out the week and day of your program—for example, Week 1, Day 1— as well as the date.

TAKE YOUR KETO READING

Check your ketostick every morning and record the result under "Keto Reading." It may take a couple of days to achieve ketosis, which is indicated by a pink to purple color on your ketostick. If you haven't achieved ketosis by the morning of the third day, decrease your carb intake to between 50 and 60 grams. Remember that if you take in too many carbs on your Menu Days, it will knock you out of ketosis.

WEIGH YOURSELF

Weigh yourself every morning and record the result under "Weight." Try to weigh yourself at the same time every day and the same way: nude and after emptying your bladder.

PLAN TO OVERCOME TODAY'S OBSTACLES

Every morning, check your schedule for any challenging events you may encounter during the day. Make a plan to overcome these challenges and write it down under "Plan to Overcome Today's Obstacles."

CHOOSE YOUR AFFIRMATIONS

Write down one or two positive statements under "Affirmation" that you will repeat to yourself throughout the day. For more information on how affirmations can help you become Lean for Life, see Day 17 in Chapter 6.

TRACK YOUR MEALS AND FLUIDS

Jot down *everything* you eat and drink, *every time* you eat or drink, and do it immediately after every meal, snack or beverage. We've all experienced cases of "food fog," when we forget about that handful of candies we ate out of the bowl on the receptionist's desk as we headed back to our office after lunch, which is why it's so important to write things down right away. Studies show that the longer you wait, the more likely you are to make an error. Under "Time," indicate the time of day for all your meals and snacks. Be sure to include the serving sizes of everything you consume under "Serving Size." On your Protein Days, you'll be tracking how many grams of protein you consume at each meal and snack (under "Carbs") and adding up the total for each day. On your Menu Days, it's the carbs you'll be tracking (under "Carbs grams"). *Remember, before you eat anything on your Menu Days, know how many carbs it contains.* Under "Water," add up the total number of ounces of fluids you have consumed. We recommend a minimum of 80 ounces of water or other calorie-free beverages per day.

TAKE YOUR VITAMINS

Take your Lean for Life vitamins and mineral supplements (or an equivalent) and write down the time of day you took them under "Vitamin."

TRACK YOUR ACTIVITIES

Under "Activities/Durations," jot down all the physical activity you do throughout the day, including the type of activity and duration. And yes, things like taking the stairs at work and doing housework count!

RECORD YOUR TOTAL NUMBER OF STEPS

On this program, you're encouraged to use a pedometer, an accelerometer or other device to track the number of steps you take every day. Write down your total number of steps for the day under "# Pedometer Steps."

USE YOUR SUCCESS LEARNING TOOLS

On a daily basis, you'll be making use of a number of tools that are designed to enhance your success, such as reading this book, using the Lean for Life online program, and more. Record the tools you use each day under "Success Learning Tools."

TAKE YOUR BODY MEASUREMENTS ONCE A WEEK

See chapter 3 (page 54) for instructions on how to take your measurements and record them under "Body Measurements."

TAKE NOTES

Under "Notes," jot down anything else that you think is important, such as your moods, levels of hunger or satiety, surprising insights, or just a few encouraging words to keep you motivated or to congratulate yourself for a job well done. You deserve it!

View DAP sheets.

The Inside Story from Dr. Allouche

PUT YOUR METABOLISM ON "PAUSE"?

Your Protein Days act like a shock to your system that hits the "pause" button on your metabolism. Don't worry, putting your metabolism on pause is a good thing, and here's why. In a lean, healthy body, metabolism converts food to fuel for energy, stores some fuel in your fat cells for later use and burns fat as needed to help keep you lean. It's as if your metabolism is on cruise control and you're flying through life in the fast lane. But when you're overweight, your metabolism gets out of whack.

Think of your body like a sleek SUV. If you fill it up with premium fuel and keep it free of any junk, it will get the best gas mileage possible and can speed down the highway for miles and miles. But if you fill up the tank with cheap gas and overload every square inch of the trunk with bowling balls, then your gas mileage is going to suffer. Keep stuffing more bowling balls on the rear seats, the passenger seat, and even the roof of the vehicle, and eventually something's gotta give. You can no longer keep up with the cars in the fast lane, and you risk breaking a shaft or blowing a tire.

It's the same scenario for your body, which can only metabolize so much food. When you're eating too much or eating too many of the wrong kinds of foods, your metabolism gets overloaded just like your SUV. It has to work harder than ever to keep up with all the food that's coming in, converting more of it to energy to keep your larger body operating, shoveling more of it into your fat cells for storage and trying to burn some of that fat. Over time, your metabolism becomes inefficient, and it can no longer handle all its duties. Can you guess which is the first function that falls to the wayside? Fat burning.

THE FALLOUT FROM OVERTAXING YOUR METABOLISM

One of the problems associated with a metabolism that's gone haywire involves insulin. As you saw in chapter 1, after you eat, carbohydrates are broken down into simple sugars and released into the bloodstream. It's insulin's job to clear glucose out of the bloodstream and to guide it into your body's cells. Some of that glucose heads to the liver, where it is converted into *glycogen* that can be used by the muscles. The rest of the glucose that isn't used by your body's cells, about 30 percent, is ushered into your fat cells to be stored as fuel for use at a later time.

When you're eating too much, and especially eating too many carbohydrates, your insulin production rises. When insulin levels are high, a greater percentage of glucose heads straight into your fat cells, causing them—and your waistline—to swell. This process of converting food into fat is called *lipogenesis*, and it occurs in direct relation to the level of insulin secretion. The more insulin you're producing, the more fat you're creating.

THE INSULIN-CARB CONNECTION

When you eat too many refined carbs, your blood sugar levels soar, triggering the release of a surge of insulin that works overtime to clear the glucose out of your bloodstream. The problem is that insulin does such a good job that it clears out too much glucose and your blood sugar level drops below optimum. Low blood sugar levels lead to cravings for more sweets and refined carbs, so you indulge again, causing another burst of insulin production. This effectively puts you on a blood sugar roller coaster of cravings, spikes and crashes.

Eventually, if you nibble on sweets throughout the day to satisfy your cravings, your insulin production mechanism gets stuck in the "on" position, with insulin being released almost constantly. After years of overproducing insulin, your body can become resistant to its effects, and the glucose remains in your bloodstream rather than being cleared out. This is called insulin resistance, and it can lead to pre-diabetes or full-blown type 2 diabetes, as well as excess weight.

HOW HITTING THE "PAUSE" BUTTON REVERSES THE PROBLEM

To get your overloaded metabolism back in working order, you need to slow it down temporarily by limiting your carbohydrate and fat intake and reducing calories. This puts the pause on your metabolism; then you hit the switch and turn it back on again. It's kind of like resetting your modem when your internet connection goes on the fritz—you have to unplug it and let it remain off for a short time; then you plug it back in and turn it on again.

With this program, your Protein Days are designed to put your metabolism on pause by limiting carbohydrate and fat intake and reducing calories. This is why it is so important that you stick with the recommended proteins on these days. Then the foods you'll be eating on your Menu Days help fire it back up and—voilà!—your metabolism eventually starts burning fat so your fat cells can start shrinking.

Dr. Stamper Says

THE SIX ESSENTIALS—ESSENTIAL #1: MAKE IT YOUR GOAL TO *LEARN* TO BE LEAN FOR LIFE.

You're probably familiar with the saying: "It's not about the destination; it's about the journey." That couldn't be more true when it comes to getting and staying lean. Most diets are all about the destination, which is why they don't work for the long term. They only focus on short-term changes in dietary composition, and when the diet ends, so does the weight loss—at least for most people.

With Lean for Life, the focus is on the journey—*learning* what it takes to become lean as you shrink your fat cells so you will be able to stay lean long after you've completed the program. The learning process begins today. As you learn more on each day of this program, you'll create new neural connections within your brain. By practicing what you're learning each and every day of this program, you'll strengthen those new connections and, eventually, making healthy choices will seem like second nature.

DAY 2: PROTEIN DAY

DO YOU HAVE A TOUCH OF THE "DIET FLU"?

When I (Cynthia) was 17, I was Dr. Stamper's guinea pig. In order to help me lose a few pounds, he put me on the diet that would evolve into the Lean for Life program you're doing now. On my second day on the diet, I woke up feeling out of sorts. I complained to my mom that I was tired, I had a headache, and I just didn't feel good. "Something's wrong with me," I whined. My mom just smiled, patted me on the head, and assured me I'd feel better in a day or so. And she was right. Just a couple of days later, I not only felt better, I felt great!

**EAT BETTER
MOVE MORE
STRESS LESS**

Today is the second day of your three initial Protein Days. To achieve ketosis, aim for about 50 to 80 grams of carbohydrates.

Today, hundreds of thousands of patients later, I understand that what I had was a case of what we call the "diet flu." This isn't a real flu or illness, but when you first restrict calories and carbohydrates, you may experience temporary food withdrawal symptoms that make you feel like you're under the weather or just a little "off." If this happens to you, don't be alarmed. It's perfectly normal for your body to react whenever you make significant changes in the way you eat. Not everybody gets the diet flu, but if you do, understand that, like my mom said, it's only temporary and you should feel better soon.

One of the best passages I've seen on food withdrawal symptoms comes from a book called *Forever Thin* by Theodore Isaac Rubin, M.D. In discussing food addiction, Dr. Rubin explains that when a person's "normal" food supply is in any way curtailed, the individual may experience both physical and psychological reactions that can vary in degree and are sometimes mistaken for other illnesses. Rubin writes, "There may be digestive, respiratory, urinary, circulatory, and emotional disturbances in any number of combinations."

So what can you do to cope with the diet flu? First, this is a good time to come to grips with the fact that changing your eating habits may be uncomfortable at times and that getting through your first few Protein Days may present a challenge. Let's call it a reality check. If you can accept that you may have to deal with some brief internal discomfort in order to achieve ketosis and start burning fat, you'll greatly increase your chances for success on the program. Second, take comfort in knowing that there are many quick fixes that can alleviate symptoms of the diet flu. In the following section, you'll find some of the more common symptoms our patients report and what you can do if you experience them.

DIET FLU REMEDIES

GOT A CASE OF THE DIET FLU?

Be sure to eat at least 50 grams of carbohydrates—but no more than 80 grams!—on your Protein Days to minimize diet flu symptoms. Consuming some of the dairy choices from the approved "Lean Foods" list in chapter 2 and eating some of the high PER protein products can help increase your carb intake.

FEELING HUNGRY?

You may need to eat more protein servings and have more high PER protein snacks throughout the day. Be sure to keep extra protein snacks on hand in case you need them. If you're reaching the high end of the carb range for ketosis (near 80 grams per day), choose lower-carb snacks.

HAVE A HEADACHE?

If your head is pounding, your first reaction may be to reach for the aspirin, ibuprofen or acetaminophen. But there are other solutions. Consuming at least 50 grams of carbs per day can help prevent or reduce headaches. In addition, don't wait too long between snacks and meals. Most people feel best when eating a protein snack about every two hours. Low sodium (salt) levels, which can occur when you restrict carbs, are another cause of headaches. Adding table salt to your food or drinking two cups of prepared bouillon a day can help. (If you have high blood pressure, check with your physician before increasing your salt intake.) Another culprit that causes headaches is caffeine withdrawal. If you choose to decrease your caffeine intake, do so gradually to minimize the possibility of headaches. Mild dehydration is another cause of headaches so make sure you're drinking enough fluids.

FEELING LIGHTHEADED OR DIZZY, ESPECIALLY WHEN STANDING?

Mild dehydration or low sodium levels may be to blame. Drink more fluids, and as long as you don't have high blood pressure, you may need to add salt to your diet or drink a cup of bouillon twice a day during the Rapid Weight Loss phase of the program.

EXPERIENCING MUSCLE WEAKNESS, CRAMPING OR GENERAL MUSCLE FATIGUE?

These symptoms can be a sign of mild dehydration or low potassium. Make sure you're drinking enough water and getting enough potassium. Most of our patients report that they feel best when they take three—or more, if needed—over-the-counter potassium tablets every day, in addition to their vitamins. You can purchase potassium at most drugstores, health food stores and grocery stores.

FEELING CONSTIPATED?

In some people, dieting can lead to constipation, which is often caused by mild dehydration. The first step in preventing and resolving constipation is to increase your daily fluid intake. Squeezing a little lemon juice in your water is a simple trick that may help alleviate constipation. Taking a natural fiber supplement can also be helpful. If you experience frequent constipation, you may want to try either sugar-free Metamucil or Citrucel three times a day. You may also want to try the Lean for Life fiber supplement products. If you need more help, you can try Colace, an over-the-counter stool softener. In more extreme cases, you could try a glycerin suppository or a laxative like milk of magnesia.

HAVE HEARTBURN OR INDIGESTION?

Over-the-counter antacids may relieve the temporary heartburn or indigestion associated with changing your eating habits. Another simple strategy is to add one quarter of a teaspoon of baking soda to a glass of water every morning.

HAVE "KETO-BREATH"?

During weight loss, ketones (the by-product of fat burning) are excreted through your breath as well as through the urine. In some people, this can cause unpleasant breath. Here's what you can do to combat "keto-breath":

- Chew sugarless gum.
- Use breath spray.
- Keep your mouth moist by sipping water throughout the day.
- Add a thick, fresh lemon slice to your water and feel free to chew a bit of the lemon rind.
- Chew a sprig of fresh parsley.
- Take chlorophyll capsules (one brand recommends taking 90 to 100 milligrams a day, usually at night).

The Inside Story from Dr. Allouche

WHAT'S REALLY BEHIND THE DIET FLU?

The diet flu may be due to fluctuating blood sugar levels that can occur when carbs are suddenly restricted. If you're like many of our patients who have spent years consuming too many carbs, reducing your carb intake can act like a shock to your system. Here's how.

As you saw in chapter 1, eating too many carbs increases insulin production. The amount of insulin secreted is directly related to the amount of glucose derived from your food—the higher the carb content, the more glucose in your bloodstream and the more insulin released. (Check out the Glycemic Index Chart in Appendix C to see the impact various foods have on the amount of glucose in your bloodstream.) When you consume too many carbs over years or decades, it leads to chronically higher levels of blood sugar and insulin. The problem here is that your body burns that abundance of glucose for fuel and never gets around to burning the fat stored in your fat cells. So your fat cells keep getting, well, fatter. As you read earlier, creating more fat is known as lipogenesis.

Restricting carbs and being in ketosis is the key to reversing this trend. Over time, being in ketosis lowers blood sugar and insulin levels, helps rebalance insulin receptors on your cells to enhance insulin sensitivity and retrains your body to burn fat for fuel, which is called *lipolysis*. Be aware that it can take time for your body to remember how to use the contents of your fat cells for energy, causing them to shrink in size. How quickly your body starts burning and shrinking fat cells depends in part on the amount of excess weight you're carrying around. If you have 100 pounds to lose, it may take a bit longer than if you have only 20 pounds to lose.

Be aware that during this adjustment period, your body may feel like it's desperately seeking energy. Without its usual source of fuel—glucose—and without the ability to access the contents of those plump, juicy fat cells, it can lead to fluctuating blood sugar levels that produce the symptoms linked to the diet flu.

Rest assured: as long as you aren't an insulin-dependent diabetic, temporary fluctuations in blood sugar aren't a medical emergency, and you don't need to race to the nearest vending machine for a candy bar to alleviate your symptoms. Use the simple strategies outlined above to help prevent or reduce the severity of any symptoms you may experience. And in a few days, you'll stop feeling "blah" and start feeling fantastic.

DAY 3: PROTEIN DAY

REPTILIAN REVENGE

Did you know that nearly 45 percent of our everyday actions are habits that involve little to no decision-making? As you'll see in today's "Inside Story from Dr. Allouche," you can thank—or blame—the most ancient part of your brain, known as the reptilian brain, for these automatic behaviors. We have seen with our patients that it is often these mindless habits that are contributing to weight gain. And the key to better health is changing these habits.

Changing your habits can be challenging. Change takes effort, and it makes you uncomfortable. It may even frighten you. Don't be surprised if you find yourself resisting change during this program. In fact, expect it. It's a completely normal part of the process. Attempts to change are almost always met with some inner resistance. Why? When you try to adopt new habits, your brain fights back because it is hardwired to prefer routine.

EAT BETTER MOVE MORE STRESS LESS

Today is the last of your three initial Protein Days. Are you in ketosis yet? Whether or not you have achieved ketosis, begin your first Menu Day tomorrow on Day 4.

It may not be easy to change, but it's not impossible. For more than 40 years, we have been helping patients overcome that inner resistance and successfully trade in their old, self-destructive habits for new, healthy ones. Here are some of the most effective tips and strategies that have helped our patients and that can help you to make the changes necessary to become Lean for Life.

ADOPT A CAN-DO ATTITUDE

Research shows that if you believe your actions can change your life, you're more likely to engage in the healthy habits that will help you lose weight. If you think that your destiny is controlled by fate or luck, you aren't as apt to adopt good-for-you behaviors. Based on the success of so many of our patients who have changed their habits and changed their lives for the better, it's clear that the little choices you make on a daily basis can make a big difference in your life. So start believing in your ability to control your own destiny. Consider the following for today's affirmations:

I can change my habits.

I am in control of my own destiny.

TAKE IT ONE STEP AT A TIME

Now that you have made the decision to become Lean for Life, you probably want it to happen *right now*! But we have found that the people who are the most successful at changing their behavior are the ones who do so gradually. Remember, the habits—and the excess weight—you have now didn't appear overnight. They developed over time, and it will take time to change them.

I want to tell you about a friend of mine. He's completed every marathon he has ever entered. His strategy is simple. "Focus on the steps," he says, "and the miles take care of themselves." If you think about it, this strategy applies in many areas of life. It certainly does with weight loss.

Rather than becoming overwhelmed by the 20, 50 or 75 pounds you want to lose, start your journey one step at a time. Try focusing every day on those small decisions you can make that will move you one step closer to a healthy weight. One less soft drink, one more glass of water. One less escalator, one more set of stairs. One less TV show, one more walk around the block. Over time, these seemingly small changes add up to noticeable results. It's been said that a journey of a thousand miles begins with a single step. Why not take a step or two today toward the weight, the body and the health you desire?

NON-FOOD REWARDS

Enjoy time alone.

Engage in your favorite activity.

Relax in a bubble bath.

Read a favorite book.

Browse through your favorite magazine.

Treat yourself to a manicure and/or pedicure.

Get a massage.

Get a facial.

Listen to music.

Treat yourself to some new exercise gear.

Spend time with friends or family.

Make or buy a piece of fun jewelry.

Buy a colorful scarf.

Participate in your favorite hobby.

Go window shopping.

Try a new cologne or perfume.

Get a book with blank pages and make it your "Reward Book" by writing down a compliment in it every time you make a healthy change.

Share your success through social media.

FORGIVE, BUT DON'T FORGET

If you get off track one day and revert back to your old habits, don't beat yourself up about it. Straying from your healthy new behaviors doesn't mean you're a failure or that you have to throw in the towel completely. Just get back on track as soon as possible. It's also a good idea to go over your DAP for the past few days to see what may have led you astray and make a plan to prevent or deal with a similar situation in the future.

REPLACE OLD HABITS WITH NEW ONES

Instead of trying to simply eliminate unhealthy habits, replace them with new routines. If you usually have indulgence foods immediately after dinner, start taking your dog for an after-dinner walk or use that time to write in your journal, complete your DAP or practice some form of mental training, which you'll be learning more about throughout the book. Creating new habits takes the focus away from what you're missing and shines a light on the positive benefits you're getting from your transformation.

GIVE YOURSELF A PAT ON THE BACK

It's important to reward yourself for making progress in your efforts to change your habits. If you make it an entire day without drinking a soda, or you go for a brisk walk every single day for a week, celebrate! The key is learning how to reward yourself without food. KL is a successful Lean for Lifer and a regular participant in our online chats. One of her tips for success is that she never thinks of food as a "reward." KL says, "Food is not a reward...it's fuel (for my body)." See the "Non-Food Rewards" list on page 77.

The Inside Story from Dr. Allouche

THE RESISTANT REPTILE IN YOUR BRAIN

Your brain stem, the area at the back of the brain that connects to the spinal cord, is known as your *reptilian brain*. Your reptilian brain is the most primitive region of your brain, and it is something you have in common with reptiles that have roamed the earth for millions of years. Your reptilian brain is responsible for regulating unconscious, automatic processes in your body, such as breathing, keeping your heart beating regularly, and signaling hunger and thirst.

Your reptilian brain is very powerful, and it is a creature of habit, a slave to routine. It likes to automate your behaviors so the other parts of your brain don't have to consciously think about them anymore. This helps your brain become more efficient and gives the other areas of your cortex–the biggest part of your brain–the ability to better handle all the other pressing things in your life, such as figuring out your taxes, finishing that huge project at work or helping your kids with their algebra homework.

The problem is that once your reptilian brain has automated a behavior–whether it's something good for you, such as brushing your teeth first thing in the morning or strapping on your seatbelt every time you get in the car, or something that doesn't serve you, such as gorging on fattening foods every time you get stressed or grabbing unhealthy fare every morning on your way to work–it's very hard to "un-automate" that behavior. Your reptilian brain sees these everyday habits as essential tools for your survival, even if they are actually harming your health and making you fat. This is one of the reasons why it's so hard for you to change your habits.

Any change, even a positive one like eating healthier, can be perceived as a threat to your reptilian brain's survival. Imagine that you have a pet alligator and every day for several years, you feed it large quantities of raw meat. But one day, you run out of fresh meat so you toss a couple of boiled potatoes into your gator's mouth. Do you think your gator's going to be satisfied with a few measly potatoes? No way. That gator's going to be thrashing around and angrily snapping its powerful jaws at you. If you don't get that gator some raw meat soon, it could mean trouble.

A similar scenario is happening inside your head. When you go from your old patterns of eating too much of the wrong foods to a diet focused on healthy foods that will make you leaner, your reptilian brain fights back and cries out as if you hadn't fed it at all. If you typically eat a lot of sweets and you suddenly cut sugar out of your diet, your reptilian brain will go on an all-out assault. It will be utter chaos inside your head and body. You can trick your alligator into thinking that you're giving it what it's used to getting by choosing some of the convenience foods recommended on this program. Don't feel like you're being weak if you rely on these to help get you through these first days and weeks of the program. They are designed to help ease the transition to a new way of eating and will help turn that raging alligator in your brain into a docile pet.

By sticking with this program, you will also be forcing your reptilian brain to automate new habits. Experts say it takes 21 days to create a new habit, so by the time you complete the 28-day Rapid Weight Loss component of the program, your reptilian brain may have begun automating some of your new healthy behaviors, which will help you become Lean for Life. Of course it will take more than 21 days to cement these new behaviors as lifelong habits, but you will be well on your way to making it happen. Remember, the younger you were when you picked up unhealthy habits and the longer you've been a slave to them, the more time it will take to create new, healthy lifelong habits. Be patient, and celebrate the fact that you are making progress every day.

Dr. Stamper Says

APPETITE REGULATION AND THE BRAIN

In the late 1950s, Dr. Stamper was already theorizing that the brain and satiety were largely connected with weight gain and obesity. He spent hours in a lab at the University of Mississippi Medical School, conducting experiments in an effort to understand how the brain affected appetite. These early experiments contributed to the discovery of a control center for appetite and weight loss. Histological studies showed that this center was located in the hypothalamus. These early experiences formed the foundation of Dr. Stamper's belief that there is a regulatory *setpoint* in the brain that strives to maintain a stable weight, and that if a person overeats for an extended period of time, that setpoint becomes overtaxed and resets at a higher weight, making it difficult to lose weight. The Lean for Life program is designed to help you "bypass" the setpoint to facilitate weight loss.

DAY 4: MENU DAY

FIGHTING THOSE @#%&*! CRAVINGS

Congratulations! You've made it through your initial Protein Days! You're probably feeling pumped and ready to start your Menu Days. But if you're like many of our patients, you might find that despite your best intentions, you may struggle with pesky cravings. Of course, cravings can pop up at any time, but they are especially common during the first few days and weeks of the program. In this chapter, we could describe a lot of the tempting foods that are most likely to trip you up, but we have intentionally chosen *not* to specifically name any of them. This is because our patients have informed us that just reading the name of a favorite indulgence food this early in the program can trigger a craving. Today's goal is to learn how to control your cravings, and it is one of the most important lessons you'll learn in this program.

You know how it happens. You're doing your best to follow your program—eating better, moving more and stressing less—when all of a sudden...*WHAM!* A nagging temptation for one of your favorite foods grabs hold and refuses to let go. The more you try to ignore the siren call, the more tempting it becomes. If you give in to those cravings, it can undermine your self-esteem, shake your self-confidence and derail your weight loss. What's the problem? Is it that you simply have no self-control?

The good news is that you don't have to rely on sheer willpower to resist cravings. There are a number of physical, emotional and environmental causes for cravings. Throughout this book, you'll learn how to address these root causes, and you'll discover how to prevent or reverse them so you can minimize cravings for the long term. But if you're experiencing cravings today, you need to know what you can do *right this minute* to get rid of them. Help is on the way. On this day, you'll discover a few simple strategies that can have an almost immediate effect to help you conquer those cravings, not just today but also throughout this process.

**EAT BETTER
MOVE MORE
STRESS LESS**

Today is your first Menu Day. On your Menu Days, eat all meals at their appropriate times and do not combine meals and snacks. Eating off the program can result in too many carbohydrates and/or calories at one time, and that can negatively affect your ketosis and weight-loss results.

YOUR EMERGENCY CRAVINGS TOOLKIT

Whenever your worst cravings strike, these strategies will help you strike back to keep them under control.

GET OFF THE COUCH

Did you know that as few as 10 minutes of moderate activity reduces cravings? When temptation hits, take a brisk walk.

GET NAKED

It may sound crazy, but one of our patients swears by this strategy. She says, "If you get the urge to eat one of your danger foods, take off your clothes, stand naked in front of a mirror, and see if you still want to eat it while looking at yourself. It works for me!"

DON'T SKIP MEALS OR SNACKS

When you go for long periods of time without eating, it causes your blood sugar levels to dip. That's when you're more likely to give in and gobble up the leftovers from your toddler's birthday party or whip into the drive-through lane at your favorite fast-food spot. To help keep your blood sugar levels stabilized, don't skip meals or snacks while following this program.

HIDE YOUR TRIGGER FOODS

When your favorite food is sitting right in front of you, it's very hard to resist. Eliminate temptation by hiding your trigger foods so they aren't "staring at you." Or simply throw away or give away the foods you crave most.

AVOID YOUR "DANGER ZONES"

You can bolster your self-control by avoiding places you know will prompt your cravings. If the vending machine in the office break room is your downfall, take your break outdoors. If your favorite fast-food restaurant lies in wait for you on your drive home, avoid the ambush by taking an alternate route.

Dr. Stamper Says

THE SIX ESSENTIALS—ESSENTIAL #2: LEARN TO CONTROL CRAVINGS.

Dr. Stamper tells patients that dieters don't fail because of a lack of willpower—they fail because of cravings. Although the urge to eat certain foods may seem to come out of nowhere, cravings are actually the result of various factors—**physical** (your setpoint, as explained below) **psychological** (eating when stressed, depressed, anxious or bored) and **environmental** (the concession stand at the movies, the office vending machine and so on)—all of which affect the way your brain and body function. Dr. Stamper says, "All three causes must be dealt with because a craving is dangerous to your program. **Once you understand the causes of cravings and learn the solutions for overcoming them, you'll be on your way to being Lean for Life.**"

One of the physical causes of cravings is an elevated *setpoint*. Your brain, digestive tract and body all "talk" to each other in an effort to regulate appetite and metabolism so you can maintain a stable weight. The weight your body strives to maintain is commonly known as the setpoint. Think of your setpoint as a thermostat. Just as a thermostat works to maintain a constant temperature by regulating the heating or cooling system in response to outside conditions, your setpoint raises or lowers your appetite and metabolism in response to what you're eating.

Prolonged periods of overeating can elevate the setpoint, causing your body to strive to maintain a higher weight by lowering metabolism and increasing appetite. The situation is compounded when you try to lose weight simply by eating less. Your elevated setpoint ratchets up hunger and cranks up cravings, making it very difficult to stay on a program. Ketosis allows you to "bypass" the setpoint and dramatically reduces feelings of hunger and cravings. This makes the weight loss experience more comfortable and effective.

STAY HYDRATED

When you're dehydrated, your brain may misinterpret the signal for thirst with a craving for food. Keep your water bottle handy!

SINK YOUR TEETH INTO A TASTY HIGH PER PROTEIN SNACK

Protein-based treats and snacks are one of the most powerful weapons in your arsenal in the war against cravings. When you're on the road, it's hard to keep a serving of salmon, pork tenderloin or tofu on hand without it spoiling. And frankly, when you're craving something delicious after lunch, a serving of salmon probably isn't going to satisfy you. This is where high PER protein-based convenience snacks really come in handy. Keep them in your purse, briefcase, car or desk for emergencies.

CALL A FRIEND OR OTHER LEAN FOR LIFER

Sometimes, just talking to someone about your cravings can help get the obsessive thoughts out of your head so you can go back to concentrating on other things.

Access information about coaching and support to help you with your program.

LONGER-TERM CRAVINGS SOLUTIONS

For ongoing assistance in curbing your cravings, try the following on a regular basis.

GET YOUR SHUT-EYE

Have you ever spent the night tossing and turning only to wake up feeling ravenous and craving everything in sight? Your hunger hormones are primarily regulated while you sleep, and skimping on shut-eye can throw those hormones out of whack. Getting the seven to nine hours of sleep you need each night can help you minimize cravings. Later in this book, you'll discover some of the secrets to getting the restful sleep you need.

BOOST YOUR WILLPOWER WITH THE "10-MINUTE TIME OUT"

Want to know how to pump up your willpower? You've got to practice it, and often. You can start with something called the 10-Minute Time Out. When you get the urge to check your phone messages, make yourself wait for 10 minutes before you check them. When you want to hit the "Buy" button on an online shopping site, step away from your computer for 10 minutes and then see if you still want to make that purchase. And when you get a craving for something after dinner, take a 10-minute walk and then see if you're still laser-focused on the tempting food when you return. When you first start doing this, 10 minutes may seem like an eternity. But after a while, you'll find the time flies by faster and faster. This is an indicator that your willpower is getting stronger.

TRY THE SUPPLEMENT SOLUTION

Certain nutritional supplements may help calm cravings. If you're a patient in one of our clinics, your Lean for Life coach can help guide you to the best supplement solutions for your individual needs. In general, dietary supplements that impact serotonin may be beneficial and include 5-HTP, L-tryptophan, inositol, and St. John's wort. A new supplement that is showing promise as a cravings buster is casoxine, a powder derived from peptides found in milk.

STOCK UP ON THE SUNSHINE VITAMIN

Did you know that having low levels of vitamin D has been associated with increased food cravings and weight gain? Or that 70 percent of U.S. adults have vitamin D deficiency, about the same percentage of Americans who are overweight or obese? Getting about 20 minutes a day of sunshine (without sunscreen) or taking a daily vitamin D supplement can pump up your levels. In addition, many of the foods you'll be eating on this program contain vitamin D and may help quell cravings.

On your Protein Days, choose approved proteins that are rich in vitamin D, such as salmon, tuna, pork, eggs, nonfat milk (vitamin D fortified), nonfat plain yogurt (vitamin D fortified) and fat-free Swiss cheese. On your Menu Days, you can boost your vitamin D intake with ready-to-eat cereals (look for ones that say "vitamin D fortified") and grains from the "Lean Foods" list in chapter 2 as well as mushrooms (shiitake mushrooms contain the most vitamin D).

CRAVINGS, THE REWARD SYSTEM, AND YOUR GUT

If you have a habit of giving in to uncontrollable cravings, you might want to stop blaming yourself and start pointing the finger at your brain's reward system *and* your gut.

HOW YOUR BRAIN PLAYS A ROLE

Let's look first at your brain's reward system, which includes your demanding reptilian brain. This reward system is a sophisticated network of brain regions—including areas involved with hunger and habits (your reptilian brain), satisfaction and emotional memories—critical to our survival. It also plays a major role in food addiction and cravings.

- **Hunger center:** The hunger center of your brain is located in the brain stem, which we've previously referred to as your reptilian brain. As you saw earlier, it is involved in automating your behaviors, good or bad, and is also responsible for regulating unconscious processes in your body, such as breathing and keeping your heart beating regularly.

- **Satisfaction center:** The satisfaction center of your brain, called the *nucleus accumbens*, is what drives you to engage in the pleasurable behaviors that are necessary for survival, such as eating, drinking and having sex. Whenever you do the things that keep you—and the human species—alive, you are rewarded with a dose of feel-good chemicals that make you want to repeat the behavior.

- **Emotional memory center:** The emotional memory center of your brain, called the *globus pallidus*, is where you store emotional memories tied to the rewards you get from food. Remember that treat your mother used to give you when you were feeling low? Your emotional memory center does. And it wants that good feeling again.

The reward system communicates with the brain's planning and decision-making center to compel you to *act* on its needs and wants. The planning and decision-making center of your brain, called the cortex, is where you strategize how to take action to achieve your goals and desires. Your cortex acts as "Command Central" in your brain, sending and receiving information from all the other areas of your brain and taking all that data into consideration for planning and decision-making. This is also the area of your brain that puts the brakes on bad behaviors. When it's operating properly, it gives you the power to say no to pesky foods. When it's weak, the brakes don't always work.

Back in the days before we had thousands of industrialized food products available, the reward system simply encouraged you to eat for survival. And it still does. For example, in a healthy, lean person, biting into an apple causes the reward system to dole out a dose of those feel-good chemicals for an almost immediate mood boost. The next time the brain stem sends out the hunger signals, the nucleus accumbens motivates that lean person to seek out another apple, and everybody's happy.

But the reward system can spiral out of control. Let's say you trade in that apple for something far more *délicieux*. And let's say you don't go for a petite version of the food, but rather for a jumbo, industrial-sized number. As the decadent ingredients register in your brain, your reward system spews out a massive amount of those euphoria-inducing chemicals, making you feel like you're on cloud nine.

So what do you think your nucleus accumbens is going to motivate you to eat next time? The boring apple? Not a chance. The "danger" food is going to win out every time. For some people, eating one single decadent food is enough to completely disrupt the reward system and basically become addicted. For others, it takes time and repeatedly overindulging in tempting fare to throw the system off balance.

Be aware that the food industry knows how powerful your brain's reward system is. And it takes advantage of this information to create food products that are designed to hijack your reward system and entice you to buy more and eat more. It's no wonder you develop a habit of giving in to your cravings and packing on the pounds.

If you try to lose weight by simply eliminating those particular foods from your diet, you and your brain are left feeling frustrated and unsatisfied. That's what most diets expect you to do—suck it up. And it's one of the main reasons why most diets don't work for the long-term.

HOW YOUR GUT GETS IN ON THE ACT

Research has determined that when harmful bacteria proliferate in your gut, it makes you more vulnerable to food cravings. When the urge to indulge in tempting foods hits, harmful gut microflora communicate with your brain's reward system, indicating that they will gladly aid and abet in the assimilation of fat-promoting foods: *Hey brain, you say you want something really indulgent? Great idea! Bring it on!* Consuming certain danger foods—especially refined carbs and sweets—further promotes the growth of the bad bacteria, creating an even greater imbalance in the gut and setting in motion a vicious cycle that intensifies cravings.

KETOSIS, THE CRAVINGS CUTTER

One of your greatest allies in curbing cravings is ketosis. I like to say that ketosis acts like a neurosurgeon in the brain, using an invisible scalpel to sever the link between your brain's hunger center and its satisfaction center. As you recall, your hunger center is the brain region that tells you *when* you're hungry, and your satisfaction center tells you *what* to eat. By severing the lines of communication between these two centers, you no longer hear your satisfaction center crying out for the unhealthy foods that contributed to your weight gain. You simply hear your hunger center informing you that you need fuel in the form of food. And healthy food will satisfy your hunger. That's the power of ketosis.

Ketosis also transforms your gut from an enemy into an ally in your fight against cravings. By limiting your consumption of refined carbs and sugars to achieve ketosis, you are no longer fueling the proliferation of bad bugs in your gut. This helps tip the balance of your gut bacteria in favor of the beneficial bugs that will work hard to help you get and stay lean. It takes about 21 days to rebalance your gut microflora, which is the same amount of time it takes to begin automating new habits. By the time you reach Day 21, your brain, body and gut will have gone from conspiring against you to beginning to cooperate. In the meantime, use all of the tips provided here to help you control cravings.

DAY 5: MENU DAY

KEEP MOTIVATION IN HIGH GEAR

USA Today asked 805 American adults, "What caused you to stop dieting before losing all the weight you wanted?" The top two responses? Nearly 40 percent said they got "discouraged"; 24 percent cited a "lack of interest." Sound familiar? Setting a goal is the easy part. Just ask anyone who's ever made a New Year's resolution. You begin with determination and a dream—to pay off your credit cards, to write your screenplay, to lose weight. You know what you want and vow that this time you'll make it happen. And for a while, you do what it takes.

But then something happens. Your enthusiasm ebbs. Your focus becomes fuzzy, and your determination dims. You don't give up, but you find yourself giving in. Excuses that would have never worked a week earlier are suddenly good enough. Today becomes tomorrow, and before you know it, you're back where you started, only more discouraged than before.

So how do you stick with the plan this time? Just ask any of the people whose inspiring stories are featured in this book. Every single one of them knows an important secret: your level of interest and enthusiasm directly impacts your ability to maintain your motivation and to achieve success. In other words, the more enthused, the more you lose. This concept is so fundamental to this program that it is one of Dr. Stamper's Six Essentials.

Dr. Stamper Says

THE SIX ESSENTIALS—ESSENTIAL #3: YOUR LEVEL OF INTEREST AND ENTHUSIASM WILL DETERMINE YOUR LEVEL OF SUCCESS.

The greater your interest and enthusiasm for achieving your goal, the more likely you are to achieve it. On this program, enthusiasm means taking an active role in your weight loss. Becoming leaner doesn't just happen. *You make it happen.* You make it happen with your everyday actions and behaviors. That's why it's so critical to *do* the Lean for Life program rather than just trying to "eat less" the way most diets recommend. The daily actions on this program are designed to give you positive feedback that can keep you motivated. For example:

- Test your ketostick every morning.

- Weigh yourself every morning.

- Complete your DAP every day.

- Look at your "My Motivator Cards" (page 52) several times a day.

- Repeat your Affirmations several times a day.

- Read, or re-read, *The New Lean for Life* book every day.

- Look at your "After" photo often.

- Take your measurements every week.

The Inside Story from Dr. Allouche

MEET SEROTONIN, THE MOTIVATION HORMONE

Say hello to serotonin, the happiness hormone that plays an instrumental role in keeping you motivated. This feel-good neurochemical calms stress, soothes anxiety and helps keep depression at bay—all of which help you stick with a healthy eating program. Surprisingly, your "second brain" located in your gut produces far more of your body's neurochemicals than the big brain in your head. In fact, it is estimated that about 80 percent of the body's supply of serotonin is manufactured in the gut, with only the remaining 5 percent being released directly within the brain.

The Lean for Life eating plan is designed to help heal your gut and boost serotonin. How does it do it? Ketosis. When you're in ketosis, your body produces ketones, which promote the production of serotonin. People in dietary ketosis often report increased physical and mental energy, less moodiness, less irritability and less depression. Some even say they feel euphoric while in ketosis.

Why would ketosis produce more serotonin to make you feel better? Let's look back to two of our cave-dwelling ancestors—we'll call them Caveman Krunk and Cavewoman Gurk—for a clue. Krunk and Gurk, your average Stone Age couple, had to hunt for their food, and when they were successful, they would enjoy a veritable feast. But when food was scarce and Krunk came back to the cave empty-handed, they might have to fast for several days. The fasting would trigger ketosis, which not only reduces hunger but also sparks serotonin production. In turn, this helped keep Krunk and Gurk from getting depressed about the lack of food until their next successful hunt.

When you enter into ketosis, it's like unlocking your inner caveman or cavewoman. You're basically reacquainting your body with a natural state that you are genetically programmed to experience. The boost in serotonin can keep your mood elevated while you reduce your calorie intake so you can successfully shed pounds and actually feel good while doing so.

CALM YOUR MIND TO CRANK UP THE SEROTONIN

Being in ketosis isn't the only way to increase serotonin. Calming your mind with meditation also boosts it. On Day 1, we talked about how your body and metabolism become overloaded and benefit from being put on "pause." The same thing goes for your brain. It's probably been working overtime and needs a breather, too. Meditation, and its subsequent serotonin boost, soothes stress and anxiety and wards off distracting thoughts and worries so you can focus on achieving your goals. You don't have to be an expert at meditation to see the benefits. A 2011 study from Japanese researchers found that when novices practiced a form of meditation involving deep breathing, they experienced a significant increase in serotonin in just 20 minutes. See Day 10 in chapter 5 for simple forms of meditation you can do anywhere, anytime.

HEAL YOUR GUT TO SPARK SEROTONIN PRODUCTION

If your gut is harboring an army of bad microflora, it may interfere with the production of serotonin and may be one of the reasons why you've gotten discouraged with dieting in the past. By following this program's eating plan, you can begin healing your gut, which will promote serotonin production. And when adequate levels of the neurochemical are circulating in your body, it will be easier for you to maintain your motivation to stick with your program.

DAY 6: MENU DAY

THINK ABOUT YOUR THINKING HABITS

When we hear the word "habits," most of us think solely about our actions— logging on to Facebook or Twitter first thing in the morning, or taking the same route to work day in and day out. But did you know that your thoughts can be habit-forming, too? Think about it.

When you look in the mirror, do you automatically think, *I'm so fat*.

When you think about getting fit, is your first reaction, *Ugh, I hate exercise*.

When you consider trying to lose weight, does the following pop into your head, *I always gain it back*.

The more you focus on negative thoughts, the more your brain strengthens the neuronal pathways and synapses—or connections—that support negative thinking. You're basically hardwiring your brain to stay stuck in a negative loop that doesn't bode well for your waistline. Did you know that every thought that flies through your head releases brain chemicals? Negative thoughts release chemicals that slow down your brain's ability to function and make it harder to process thoughts and problem-solve. Negative thinking is also linked to fearful feelings, which impact an area of the brain called the temporal lobe, which is involved with impulse control, the kind of control you need when faced with a box of doughnuts in the office break room. When you're bombarded by negative thoughts, you're much more likely to gobble up a glazed number, one with chocolate sprinkles, and then maybe even one of the bear claws, too.

Negative thoughts are so harmful, we call them your "inner sabotage agents." Their mission is to hold you hostage in the body you currently have and to thwart your efforts to change your habits. When you try to make healthy changes, your inner sabotage agents plant thought bombs in your head that trip you up and keep you chained to your old habits. These thought bombs can explode at any moment, even when you think you're well on your way to making lifelong changes. And the explosion can reverberate, setting off other thought bombs until your mind is completely under siege, and you're ready to wave the white flag and give up on your efforts to change your habits.

Every single day of your life, up to 50,000 thoughts race through your head. How many of your thoughts are inner sabotage agents that are holding you back? If you're like most of the patients we see, you probably have your fair share of inner sabotage agents lurking inside your head. Let's look at some of the most common types of inner saboteurs and how they plot against you.

TYPES OF INNER SABOTAGE AGENTS

"IT'S ALL OR NOTHING"

When you think in these terms, you tend to label your eating habits in extremes, so if your performance falls short of your expectations and you indulge in a not-so-healthy food, or if you don't meet all your weight-loss goals, you see yourself as a failure. Sarah, for example, went from a size 12 to a size 8 on the program, but her reaction was *I'm still too fat*. Why? Because her goal had been to get back into a size 6, which she had worn in college.

OVERGENERALIZING

When you take a single negative event or experience and apply it more broadly to your life, you are overgeneralizing. Ryan had been following his program to the letter for four full weeks and had dropped two belt notches when he went to his brother's wedding and indulged in a big piece of wedding cake. He immediately thought, *I can't follow through on anything. I'll never reach my goals, so I may as well stop trying.*

LABELING

People who tend to use labels can be brutal, especially with themselves. When Kristin found out that "move more" was one of the important pieces of the Lean for Life program, she told herself, *I'm so lazy. There's no way I can do this if I have to exercise.* The problem with labeling is that once you label yourself as "lazy," for example, you basically create a barrier that wasn't there before you thought the word.

DOOM AND GLOOM

When you see nothing but the negative side of things, you are apt to discount your successes by insisting that, for whatever reason, your achievements "don't count." You tend to hold on to negative beliefs, even when you've been contradicted by positive experiences. When Tracy lost 30 pounds on the program, she still managed to find a way to criticize herself: *My waist is a lot smaller, but it just makes my hips look bigger.*

JUMPING TO CONCLUSIONS

Jumping to conclusions, and in particular predicting the worst even though there are no facts to support such a conclusion, is one of the most self-defeating types of thinking. The problem is that when you expect the worst, you're more likely to get it. Sandra was enthusiastic about losing weight but was saddled with doubts about increasing her activity level. She thought, *My doctor told me that I have weak ankles. If I start exercising, I'm 100 percent convinced that I'll twist one of them and end up in crutches.* When Sandra went on a hike, all she could think about was tripping on a rock. She was so nervous that she kept her eyes glued to the ground the entire time and ended up hitting her head on a low branch, which caused her to stumble and—you guessed it—sprain her ankle.

BLAMING

Refusing to take responsibility for your actions and putting the blame on other people, situations and places is destructive thinking. By insisting that things are not your fault, your inner voice is also telling you that you have no control over your situation. When asked what had contributed to a 20-pound weight gain since her wedding three years earlier, Janine answered: "It's my husband's fault that I've gained weight because he's always eating sweets in front of me. How am I supposed to resist?"

DENIAL

When you won't admit that you have a problem, you certainly won't do anything to change your behavior. When our patient Debbie told a friend that she was starting the Lean for Life program and invited her to join with her so they could encourage and support one another, her friend balked: "If I get to 200 pounds, then I'll think about doing something about my weight. And even then I wouldn't need to join a program to lose weight. I could do it on my own."

RATIONALIZING

People who rationalize are experts at making excuses for their behavior. Look at Alexandra, who complained that she was doing everything possible to lose weight but still couldn't drop the pounds. When her husband opened the trunk of her car one day and found dozens of chocolate bar wrappers, she looked at him sheepishly and said, "What?! I saw a study last month saying that dark chocolate is good for you. I'm just eating it for my health." Rationalization is one of the most common stumbling blocks we see among our patients.

SILENCE YOUR INNER SABOTAGE AGENTS WITH "THOUGHT CONTROL"

With a strategy called "thought control," you can learn to take control of your thoughts and silence your inner sabotage agents. When you minimize the thought bombs in your head, it makes it so much easier to follow through with your program so you can finally get a leaner, healthier body. Here's how to do it.

LISTEN TO YOURSELF

Start paying attention to your inner sabotage agents and write down the negative thought bombs that explode in your head. You may be surprised at the volume of self-sabotage that is taking place inside your head.

TARGET THE TRIGGERS

Note the circumstances that trigger your inner saboteurs to attack. What were you doing when the barrage of negativity surged in your mind? How were you feeling? Were you hungry or tired? Look for patterns and see if you can reduce the number of negative thoughts by doing the things you need to do to prevent those situations: not skipping meals or snacks, getting adequate sleep, and so on.

IDENTIFY THE TYPE OF INNER SABOTAGE AGENTS

Do your inner sabotage agents tend to blame others for your circumstances, jump to conclusions or overgeneralize? Knowing the type of negative thoughts that are keeping you from achieving your goals can help you change them.

KNOW YOUR INNER SABOTAGE AGENT ALERT LEVEL

Become aware of the volume of negative thoughts racing through your head, and start tracking how your "alert level" impacts your eating habits.

Red: Help! I'm under attack!

Yellow: A few inner saboteurs, but I can handle it!

Green: Nothing but positive, solution-based thinking!

REPLACE NEGATIVE THOUGHTS AND MESSAGES WITH POSITIVE, SOLUTION-BASED ONES

As soon as you hear a harmful, negative message, pause and replace it with a positive or solution-based one. This may sound contrived at first, but it begins to feel more natural the more you do it. And it can have a powerful impact on your behavior. Does this mean you should lie to yourself? No, but you do need to learn to shift your perspective or the way you look at things. Look for the silver lining in negative situations and look at problems as a chance to come up with solutions to solve them. Whatever words you choose, you can counter the negative with something positive on the spot (see "Thought Control Examples").

PRACTICE

Successful weight loss involves *consistently* replacing negative thought patterns with positive new ones. To truly break self-sabotaging habits, it's important to practice more positive thinking over and over again. "Once in a while" or "every now and then" won't cut it. Mental training techniques like the ones mentioned in this section provide an opportunity to rehearse and practice positive patterns in your mind hundreds of times. This consistent repetition has a powerful influence and can lead to lasting change. Negative patterns of thought wither, and stronger patterns of self-respect and self-confidence take their place.

STOP!

Whenever your thoughts tempt you to do something that might interfere with your program, practice the method described in "STOP!" (see page 98).

THOUGHT CONTROL EXAMPLES

Inner Sabotage Agent: I hate going to the gym.

Positive, Solution-Based Thought: Even though I don't feel like exercising this morning, I know that I will feel better and have more energy after I do it. And I love the fact that I sleep better at night when I exercise.

Inner Sabotage Agent: I'm only fat because restaurants serve such big portions.

Positive, Solution-Based Thought: If I'm going to eat out, I can ask to have half my meal placed in a to-go container before they serve it to me so I won't be tempted to overeat.

Inner Sabotage Agent: I haven't lost any weight this week. I may as well quit my program.

Positive, Solution-Based Thought: If I'm not losing weight, I can try to find out why and make changes. First, I'll check my ketostick to see if I'm in ketosis. If not, I'll check my DAP for the past few days to see if I've been eating too many carbohydrates. Then I'll wrack my brain to see if I forgot to record something I ate in my DAP. If necessary, I can follow the Protein Day guidelines until I'm in ketosis again.

STOP!

Whenever you're tempted to do *anything* that might interfere with your program, **STOP!** This technique is a form of mental training that reduces impulsivity and increases your willpower.

1 STOP Visualize a stop sign and hear the word *stop*. Immediately stop what you're doing.

2 TAKE a deep breath. This creates a "window of opportunity" during which you can become aware of the temptation you're facing and can start over.

3 OBSERVE your situation, yourself and your options. What's going on? How are you feeling? Are you hungry, angry, lonely, tired? What do you want? What do you need? What really matters to you? What choices do you have? What actions will help you move toward what's really important to you?

4 PLAN your actions. Choose a plan of action based on one or more of the options available to you and put that plan into operation. Shift the focus away from food by doing something: taking a walk, calling a friend, sitting quietly for 5 minutes and letting your attention rest on your breathing, going window shopping, listening to music, working on a project or reviewing your "My Motivator Cards" to remind yourself why becoming Lean for Life is important to you.

If you find yourself thinking, *I'm tired of not eating what I want—I'm going to have a treat!* make an active choice to focus on the benefits of maintaining your plan of action. Let yourself hear whatever voices inside of you are suggesting that you abandon or sabotage your Lean for Life program, and pause long enough to acknowledge and respond to those voices. Encourage yourself as you would a close friend.

OLD WAY

FOOD, THOUGHT OR CRAVING → GIVE IN → EAT → FEEL GUILTY → GIVE UP

NEW WAY

FOOD, THOUGHT OR CRAVING → STOP! → TAKE A DEEP BREATH → OBSERVE → PLAN OF ACTION

The more often you do this, the more easily and effectively you'll be able to do it. That's because after you do something successfully again and again, it becomes hardwired in your brain, which makes it feel spontaneous and natural. It becomes part of you. It becomes a habit.

The Inside Story from Dr. Allouche

MUSCLE UP WITH PROTEIN

During both your Menu Days and Protein Days, be sure you're eating at least six protein servings a day—one each for breakfast, morning snack, lunch, afternoon snack, dinner and evening snack. If you aren't getting enough protein, you'll lose lean muscle mass, and that spells trouble for your goal of becoming Lean for Life. What do your muscles have to do with weight loss? A lot! I don't want to bog you down with too many details, but here's a quick look at the role your muscles play in the process.

Your body needs energy to perform all your daily activities—everything from breathing and pumping your blood to chasing after your toddler or running up a flight of stairs—and it gets this energy from fuel. Think of how your car needs fuel. When you go to the gas station, you can choose from "regular," "plus" or "premium." Similarly, your body can get its fuel from a variety of sources: the food you eat, your muscles or your stored fat.

Your body's number-one favorite source of energy is derived from the carbs you eat. But when you limit your carb intake, your body needs another source of energy, and it needs it *quick!* If you aren't eating enough protein, one of the first places it will turn is your muscle. When you don't get adequate protein in your diet, it means your body isn't getting all of the essential amino acids it needs to function. The body steals the amino acids from your muscles, causing them to wither away while your fat cells remain untouched. Yes, you may lose a few pounds, but instead of getting leaner, you'll look and feel weak and flabby.

Eating adequate amounts of protein ensures that your body is getting all of the amino acids it needs, which protects your muscles. This way, when carb intake is limited, the body will bypass the muscles and head to yet another energy source: your plumped-up fat cells. Burning fat to shrink your fat cells—as opposed to burning muscle—is the key to becoming lean for life. This is why it is absolutely essential that you eat at least six servings of protein while in ketosis.

DAY 7: MENU DAY

BEWARE OF INNER SABOTAGE AGENT #1: DENIAL

Welcome to Day 7! Congratulations on completing your first week! By this time, you're probably excited to be seeing and feeling some very positive changes in your body. The number on your scale should be dropping, and you may be noticing an increase in energy as well as a decrease in hunger and cravings. All of these things can help keep you motivated. It's important to understand, however, that even when you're doing well on your program, your inner sabotage agents can drop a few thought bombs in your head and derail your progress. Denial is one of the most lethal inner saboteurs, and it can be an easy trap to fall into. Even as you increase your awareness about your eating and thinking habits, you may still be in denial about some of the factors that have contributed to your weight problems. Just look at how one of our patients named Brianna struggled with denial.

Brianna and her husband, Jimmy, were big football fans, or more accurately, Chicago Bears fans. Even though the couple moved from Chicago to sunny Southern California several years ago, they still followed their Bears faithfully. Every time the Bears played during the NFL season, they would host a viewing party, replete with plenty of Chicago-style favorites. Because Brianna was trying to follow the Lean for Life program, she wouldn't partake in any of the fat-promoting fare during the game. Then, when she was cleaning up after the party, she would tell herself that since she had been so good, it was okay to have a few nibbles before she tossed the leftovers in the trash.

When she complained to us that she wasn't losing weight fast enough and wasn't in ketosis, we reviewed her DAP with her to see if we could detect any problems, but nothing seemed amiss. In talking, Brianna finally told us about the game-day tradition and admitted that she hadn't been writing down the nibbles in her DAP because she didn't think they counted as "meals" or full-fledged "snacks."

We reinforced the fact that she needed to be writing down *everything* she ate and drank in her DAP. When she did, she realized that all those little nibbles were actually adding up to a lot of calories. Now, she laughs at how she had convinced herself that "nibbles don't count" and readily admits that she was once the "Queen of Denial."

Brianna isn't alone. New research shows that people are likely to underestimate not only the number of calories they consume but also their weight. In a 2013 study appearing in *BMJ*, researchers interviewed 1,877 adults, 1,178 adolescents and 330 school-age children who dined at some of the most popular fast-food restaurants, including McDonald's, Subway, Burger King, KFC and Dunkin' Donuts. They asked the fast-food diners to estimate the calorie content of the meals they consumed. How did they do? None of the groups was even close to getting it right. The adults and kids underestimated their calorie intake by 175 calories, and the adolescents were under by 259 calories. At Lindora, we call this "portion distortion."

Our skewed perceptions also come into play when considering our own weight. Look at the results from a 2012 survey in which researchers at the University of Illinois at Urbana-Champaign asked 3,622 college students to estimate their weight in categories ranging from underweight to obese. People whose real weight fell in the normal range guessed correctly about 80 percent of the time. But nearly 60 percent of overweight students incorrectly viewed themselves as being normal weight. In the obese crowd, a whopping 90 percent underestimated their weight, believing that they were either normal weight or just overweight.

DON'T DENY IT

Denial is your number-one inner sabotage agent. Why is it so lethal? Denial protects us from painful realities. After all, as long as we're in denial, there's no problem. And if there's no problem, then there's no need to seek solutions or go through the uncomfortable process of changing our behavior. Until you understand what a destructive force denial can be, you're likely to find yourself doomed to play the no-win diet game, taking two steps forward and three steps back.

Most of us have developed a variety of ways to protect ourselves from the truth. So when we decide to make significant changes in the way we think and act, it's important that we also become aware of the hidden mental patterns that block our progress and keep us mired in those unproductive patterns and behaviors. Because we're often unaware that such patterns exist, it can be a real challenge to overcome them.

Dr. Stamper Says

THE SIX ESSENTIALS—ESSENTIAL #4: LEARN TO RECOGNIZE AND ELIMINATE YOUR DEFENSIVE BARRIERS.

Dr. Stamper refers to inner sabotage agents and other self-protective behaviors as "defensive barriers." These are ways of thinking and acting—often subconsciously—that keep you stuck in your old ways and stuck in a body you'd like to change. Defensive barriers sabotage your weight-loss efforts and impair your ability to fully integrate Essential #1: "Make it your goal to *learn* to be Lean for Life." This is why recognizing and eliminating them is one of the foundations of this program.

Two of the most common defensive barriers that impact your weight are denial and rationalization. Recognizing and disarming these particular defensive barriers can be challenging. With denial, it's a classic catch-22—in order to address a problem, you first have to acknowledge that there *is* a problem. Yet if you're deep in denial, it's unlikely that you're going to recognize or acknowledge that you are. With rationalization, we tend to use excuses to help us feel better about making unhealthy choices that don't serve our goals.

DISARMING DENIAL

Many of our patients are convinced that they don't have any real power over their lives. You may think this way, too. What you may not realize is that by making conscious changes in the way you *think*, you can change the way you *live*. It is important to remember that denial is a defense mechanism. Denial will undermine the goals you are trying to accomplish. To disarm denial, incorporate the following steps.

Take the Denial Quiz on our website to see if denial may be impacting your life.

1. Recognize denial as an inner sabotage agent and a defensive barrier.

2. Disarm denial by making a conscious decision to change the way you think and act.

3. Practice thought control on a regular basis.

By putting these skills into practice, you will gain mastery over yourself so that you are in control of your thoughts, actions and eating.

BREAK THE INSANITY CYCLE

To change the way you think, you have to break the insanity cycle. What's that? Doing the same thing over and over again and expecting a different outcome. You know, like trying the same old dieting techniques but expecting better results. That's why the Lean for Life program focuses on changing the way you think as much as the way you eat. Controlling how you think *is* controlling how you eat.

To make lasting changes, you need to gain a new awareness of how you think and how that process may be leading you down a dead-end path. See Day 6 to refresh your memory on how to combat your inner sabotage agents with thought control. Once you identify and begin eliminating those self-sabotaging thoughts that keep you stuck, you'll be one step closer to shedding those pounds and keeping them off for life.

The Inside Story from Dr. Allouche

MEASURE CHANGES INSIDE AND OUT

What are the underlying reasons why so many people are in denial about their weight? Scientists are just beginning to unravel this mystery. One theory suggests that because weight gain occurs gradually, the brain's complex software that controls self-image may not register incremental gains. Another possibility is that this software may malfunction, leading to a skewed sense of body weight. Whatever the glitch may be, it doesn't have to prevent you from achieving your goals.

To avoid denial and to encourage your new self-image, don't just rely on how you *feel* or how you *think*. Get some accurate feedback by tracking your body measurements each week. I wish there were a simple way that you could measure your fat cells as they shrink in size, but until someone invents a non-invasive, painless, inexpensive "fat cell-ometer," you'll have to rely on these body measurements:

- Weight
- Measurements of your chest, waist, lower abdomen, hips and upper-thigh area
- BMI
- Waist-to-height ratio

Taking stock of how your body is changing provides you with a valuable snapshot of the areas where you're succeeding and the areas where you could use a little more help. For this reason, it's important to give yourself a weekly progress report (see "Weekly Progress Report" in Appendix F). If you're enrolled in one of our online programs, you may be able to generate your weekly progress report with the click of a button. If not, you'll need to use your noggin, which is a good thing because your brain needs exercise, too.

Note that by following this program, you're changing more than just your external body. You're changing on the inside, too. By adopting new behaviors, you're giving your brain a good workout and are creating new neuronal pathways. By following the eating plan, you're changing the makeup of the microflora in your gut. By practicing thought control, you're changing your thinking patterns. And you're changing the way your brain, body and gut communicate with each other.

As of now, we don't have a simple way to peek inside to see these changes as they take place, but there are ways to gauge your progress. Use the "Weekly Progress Report" in Appendix F to track the intensity and frequency of your cravings, your inner sabotage agent level, your ability to practice thought control and more. This will give you a good indication of how much your brain, body and gut are changing, too.

MEASURING SHRINKING FAT CELLS

For many years in my practice in France, I've been watching my patients shrink in size when they stick to the eating guidelines described in this book. At ongoing appointments, I would typically weigh them, calculate their BMI and take their measurements. I could see their bodies getting smaller in size, but I always wondered what was happening on the inside. Their lab results told me they were getting healthier, but I wanted to see for myself. To get the answer, I teamed up with a group of researchers to investigate how an eating plan like the one you're following on Lean for Life impacts fat cells.

For this study, we tracked 13 obese people as they followed each of two four-week diets—a conventional low-calorie diet and a low-calorie diet using KOT products high in protein, high in soluble fiber, and low glycemic (similar to the Lean for Life program). The 13 participants were randomly assigned to follow one of the two diets for four weeks; then they went through an eight-week "washout" period before going on the other four-week diet.

To see how the fat cells were responding, we did what's called a needle biopsy at the beginning and at the end of each four-week diet. We used a local anesthetic on each volunteer's abdominal area, inserted a needle, and withdrew a sample of subcutaneous adipose tissue. We then examined the fat cells under a microscope.

The astounding results, which were published in the January 2012 issue of *American Journal of Clinical Nutrition*, revealed a major difference in the way fat cells reacted to the two diets. Compared to the conventional low-calorie diet, the high-protein, high-fiber, low-glycemic, low-calorie diet like the one you're following now made the *fat cells shrink twice as much in size.*

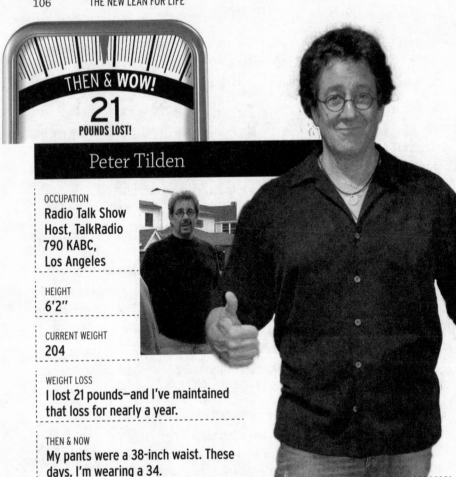

THEN & WOW!

21
POUNDS LOST!

Peter Tilden

OCCUPATION
Radio Talk Show Host, TalkRadio 790 KABC, Los Angeles

HEIGHT
6'2"

CURRENT WEIGHT
204

WEIGHT LOSS
I lost 21 pounds—and I've maintained that loss for nearly a year.

THEN & NOW
My pants were a 38-inch waist. These days, I'm wearing a 34.

The Lean for Life program gave me a sense of self-control by helping me reset my brain and change the way I think about food. I'm much more aware and conscious these days of what, when and why I'm eating. For me, that's huge!

CONQUERING CRAVINGS: The program has really helped me identify and manage my food cravings. At a party, I would knock people down to get to the cheese and bread. I never felt good after I ate it, but that never stopped me. I was addicted. Now that I've become so much more conscious of food and what triggers my cravings, it's a lot easier to stay on track and make better choices.

RECOGNIZING TRIGGERS: I used to be both a stress eater and a comfort eater, which basically meant I was eating all the time! When I was stressed,

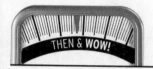

I ate. When I was relaxed or unwinding after a show, I also ate. I now realize that I ate out of habit more than hunger. Replacing old habits with healthier new ones is part of what the Lean for Life program did for me.

LEADING BY EXAMPLE: It seems as though half of my friends are dealing with some sort of serious health problem. If they don't have out-of-control blood pressure or sky-high cholesterol numbers, they're pre-diabetic or textbook candidates for a stroke. They're popping pills for this condition or that ailment. That's not how I want my future to look. I've encouraged many of my friends—and even more of my listeners—to do the Lean for Life program. I've really enjoyed seeing the positive changes that people are creating in their lives.

PLANNING AHEAD PAYS: I've been on the air for more than 20 years, and it seems like every radio station I know of has a lunchroom with a vending machine full of junk food. The sad thing is that those machines are often close to empty because people will eat anything when they get overly hungry—and that happens if you don't plan ahead. I used to be one of those guys. Now I take a cooler with me to the station. If I'm hungry during the news or commercial breaks, I munch on some celery dipped in salsa or radishes, bell peppers and a little hummus—and I never gain weight. A little advance planning really pays off.

TAKING CONTROL: There's nothing more depressing than that bloated feeling you get after you overeat. I just hate that. It's a reminder that I've lost control. There are so few things in life over which we have true control, and how we eat is one of them. The Lean for Life program gave me the tools to take responsibility for something that really matters, namely my health. It has made it possible for me to live a better life—and hopefully a longer one!

5 RAPID WEIGHT LOSS WEEK 2:

TAKE CONTROL OF YOUR BRAIN, BODY AND GUT TO STRESS LESS, FEEL HAPPIER AND PROMOTE FAT BURNING

You've successfully completed Week 1. Congratulations! By now, you should be pretty comfortable with the basics of this program—filling out your Daily Action Plan (DAP), sticking with the menu plans and curbing cravings thanks to your Emergency Cravings Toolkit. This week, we'll be introducing you to a very powerful concept called BioMod that you can use to start gaining control of your brain, body and gut to reduce stress, perk up blue moods and speed fat burning.

DAY 8: PROTEIN DAY

JOIN THE BIOMOD SQUAD

Carl, 47, was in the hospital awaiting a heart transplant when the nurse did something that made him so mad, he yelled and screamed and turned red in the face. This wasn't the only physical response to the outburst. His heart rate quickened, his blood pressure shot up and a cascade of potentially harmful physiological processes took place inside his body. The emotional upheaval took such a toll on his body chemistry that Carl was forced to wait an additional three days for his body to return to normal before undergoing surgery to get his new heart. Carl's story illustrates just how powerful the link between the mind—or rather the *brain*—and the body can be.

Over the years, our understanding of the amazing brain-body connection has deepened, and as explained earlier (see Prep Day 3 in chapter 3), we are now beginning to see that it's actually a brain-body-gut connection. We're beginning to understand how your gut microflora also influence your brain and emotions. As you've already seen, the bugs in your gut communicate with your brain to regulate or deregulate your appetite and to calm or increase cravings. Emerging research, including a 2013 study from a team of scientists at UCLA, shows that your gut bacteria also play a role in regulating your emotions, moods, cognition and even mental health, all of which can impact eating habits and, ultimately, the size of your waist. This new research provides further evidence that the lines of communication between the brain and the gut go both ways.

Together, the brain-body-gut connection, as you can see in "The Brain-Body-Gut Loop," forms a loop that can either keep your mind and body primed for weight loss or stall your efforts.

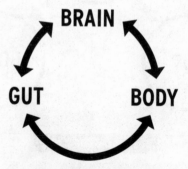

THE BRAIN-BODY-GUT LOOP

Your brain, body and gut either conspire to keep you
fat or work together to keep you lean.

The good news is that it has become even more clear that through your actions, you can *intentionally* change your brain chemistry and mental state, your body, and your gut. At Lindora, we teach a concept we call BioMod that shows you how to intentionally change your mental state, your brain biochemistry and your gut bacteria to help them go from being *less* productive to being *more* productive.

To accomplish this, you need to use BioModifiers. What are they? Very simply, they are any habit, activity, experience or ingestible that impacts your brain, body or gut. All of the BioModifiers recommended in this program provide a positive influence on your brain, body and gut that will help you shrink fat cells faster. (See "How BioMods Work.")

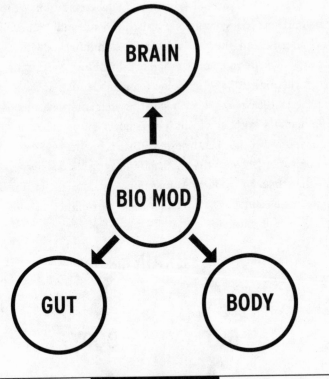

HOW BIOMODS WORKS

BioModifiers *intentionally* affect your brain, body and gut.

Check out the following lists of physical and mental BioModifiers, several of which we'll cover in more detail in this chapter's description of Rapid Weight Loss Week 2 and throughout the program.

PHYSICAL BIOMODIFIERS

- **Being in ketosis:** By being in ketosis, you're directing your brain to signal your body to increase its fat-burning capacity. Being in ketosis also helps rebalance gut bacteria to minimize cravings and potentially promote a healthier mental state.

- **Consuming probiotics:** *Probiotics* are friendly bacteria found in foods that reduce the growth of harmful gut bacteria. In 2013, UCLA researchers found that women who consumed probiotics in the form of yogurt showed changes in brain function in a variety of regions, including areas involved in emotion and cognition.

- **Exercising:** Engaging in exercise stimulates your brain's ability to produce feel-good chemicals, such as endorphins (we like to refer to them as "Leandorphins"!), and signals your muscle cells to make structural changes that increase fat-burning and carbohydrate metabolism.

- **Sleeping:** Getting adequate sleep allows your brain to balance the production of your appetite hormones and keep your metabolism running at optimal speed.

- **Listening to music:** For decades, we have known that listening to music soothes stress. Less stress means your brain releases fewer of the stress hormones that are associated with weight gain.

- **Breathing deeply:** Deep breathing is one of the fastest and most effective ways to calm stress, which also causes your brain to decrease production of the stress hormones that make you fat.

MENTAL BIOMODIFIERS

- **Thought control:** As you learned on Day 6 in chapter 4, silencing your inner sabotage agents with thought control combats negative thinking. Studies show that negative thinking causes negative changes in brain activity. Eliminating negative thoughts and replacing them with positive ones promotes positive changes in brain activity that make it easier for you to stick with your program.

- **Positive affirmations:** The positive affirmations you are repeating to yourself throughout your day are mentioned in chapter 2 and more fully described in Day 17 in chapter 6. They help shift your thought patterns from negative to positive.

- **Mental rehearsal:** Did you know that the brain makes no distinction between physical practice and mental rehearsal, when mental rehearsals are done properly? Mentally rehearsing how you will react in situations can help ensure that you will be able to do so successfully.

- **Visualizations:** Studies indicate again and again that visualizing yourself the way you want to be helps your mind to believe that it is possible to achieve that state of being.

In other words, we believe that when you train the brain, the body and gut will follow. When practiced consistently, mental rehearsals can help you enhance your performance in many areas of your life and especially in your goal to become lean. Now you try it.

- Enjoy a 10-minute nap.
- Put on your favorite music and dance.
- Take a 10-minute walk outside in the sunshine.
- Read a favorite book.
- Take a time out and breathe (see Day 10 in this chapter for a relaxing breathing exercise).
- Write down 10 positive affirmations and read them aloud.

SAY "OM" FOR BETTER HUNGER AND SATIETY SIGNALS

We've noticed that many of our patients can no longer recognize the physical signs of hunger or satiety, and this contributes to overeating. If you've lost touch with your body's appetite signals, you can get reacquainted with them by practicing a form of meditation. Before you eat anything, sit quietly for a few minutes and listen to your body. Are you really hungry? What signs of hunger do you notice—stomach growling, an empty feeling in your stomach, a feeling of weakness? On a scale of 1 to 10 (1 being not hungry at all and 10 being starving), rate how hungry you are.

As you eat, try to notice the signs of satiety. These may include a loss of interest in eating or a sense of pleasant fullness. Simple ways to increase satiety include eating more slowly, putting your fork down after every bite, chewing your food more thoroughly (at least 30 to 40 times per bite!) and eating foods that are filling, such as protein and high-fiber vegetables and fruits.

The Inside Story from Dr. Allouche

HAVE YOUR SATIETY SIGNALS GONE MIA?

When your brain, body and gut stop communicating effectively, it wreaks havoc with your *satiety*, the pleasant feeling of fullness that comes—or at least, that is supposed to come—from eating. In today's society, so many of us are eating more and more calories but feeling less and less satisfied. Why? Human physiology hasn't evolved much since the days of our cave-dwelling ancestors. Our diets and the food landscape, on the other hand, have changed drastically, especially in the last 200 years since the Industrial Revolution.

In the past, our ancestors had to make a concerted effort to go out and look for food. Now, we're constantly barraged with signals that encourage us to eat—restaurants on every corner, TV commercials for snack foods blaring all day long, boxes of doughnuts and bagels in the breakroom at work, popcorn and candy at the concession stands at the movies, hot dog vendors at the ball park and a veritable abundance of tasty treats in our own kitchens. The endless exposure has had a profound effect on the way we eat. We no longer eat only when the body tells us that we are hungry; we eat food *because it's there*. We eat food because *it's a habit*. And we don't stop eating when we are full because the body's satiety signals are on the fritz. There are three scenarios that show different types of satiety communication breakdowns based on where they originate:

- The mouth.
- The gut.
- The fat cells.

MOUTH SATIETY

As you saw in the description of pizza digestion in chapter 1, your mouth relies on a variety of flavors, smells and textures to send satiety signals to the brain. In general, a balanced amount of variety in your diet is critical for your brain, body and gut health—not enough variety can lead to imbalances in your gut microflora, yet too much variety can lead to overeating. The greater the variety of flavors, smells and textures included in a meal or a morsel of food, the more your mouth wants to sample them all. Decades of research have shown that the more food choices you have, the more calories you consume overall—call it the curse of the all-you-can-eat buffet. Eating foods that combine a variety of tastes and textures can also lead to overeating. Think of a peanut butter and bacon milkshake. Your mouth has to discern all the competing flavors and textures, including the smooth and sweet ice cream, the salty peanut butter and the crispy bacon bits.

If you're in the habit of indulging in outrageous food combinations or in tasting everything at the buffet, it may lead to problems with mouth satiety. It may take longer for your mouth to transmit satiety signals to the brain, or your mouth may no longer send them at all. For example, people who are binge eaters report that they can eat massive quantities of food without even tasting or deriving any pleasure from what they're eating.

To help you overcome problems with mouth satiety, this program structures the quantities of food you'll be eating and limits your food choices to those on the "Lean Foods" list in chapter 2 during Rapid Weight Loss.

GUT SATIETY

Based on the quantities and types of food being pulverized in the stomach, the gut sends out hormonal signals of satiety, such as cholecystokinin (CCK), peptide YY (PYY) and glucagon-like peptide 1. It sends these messages via the *vagus nerve*, which runs from your abdomen to your brainstem in an attempt to say, *Lots of food in here, you can stop eating now.* But in some people, the signaling mechanism doesn't work. The malfunction may occur because the types of food you're eating don't trigger the release of the satiety chemicals, so your gut never sends any messages to your brain. In some cases, the brain blocks all messages emanating from the digestive tract.

There's another satiety-related hormone at play in gut satiety: ghrelin. Ghrelin is the hunger hormone that makes your stomach growl and stimulates your appetite. Before mealtime, your stomach releases ghrelin and communicates with the appetite center located in the hypothalamus to encourage you to eat: *Let's go get a salad for lunch.* Skipping meals ramps up the amount of ghrelin and instead of calmly communicating with your brain, it starts screaming: *C'mon already! Let's go grab a double cheeseburger, fries and a shake! Now!*

After you've eaten, levels of ghrelin are supposed to decrease, reducing feelings of hunger. But it doesn't always work that way. Emerging evidence shows that ghrelin contributes to the reward-driven eating you learned about on Day 4 in chapter 4 that leads to cravings and dulls satiety. Having high levels of the hormone makes high-calorie foods, such as cake, chocolate and pizza, look even more tempting than when ghrelin levels aren't elevated.

Ghrelin can sabotage your weight-loss efforts in other ways, too. The hunger hormone communicates with other regions of the brain, sending messages that encourage the accumulation of visceral fat in the abdomen. This type of fat is associated with a greater risk for fatty liver, insulin resistance and metabolic syndrome—all of which make it more difficult to lose weight. In some people, weight loss sparks a marked rise in ghrelin secretion, increasing hunger to such a degree that they eat everything in sight and regain all the weight they lost.

If you have intense cravings for cakes, cookies or pizza, or if you have a habit of yo-yo dieting—losing weight but then feeling so deprived that you over-eat and gain it all back—it may be ghrelin that's driving your behavior.

The Lean for Life program offers a variety of solutions to problems with gut satiety. The protein-based foods you're eating while on this program prompt the release of the hormonal signals of satiety while keeping ghrelin in check. The high-protein convenience foods recommended on this program outsmart your biology to provide the pleasure of rewarding foods without the biological consequences. Later, you'll see how the Metabolic Adjustment phase helps prevent post-weight loss increases in ghrelin so you can avoid regaining the weight you've lost.

FAT CELL SATIETY

What do your fat cells have to do with satiety? It may be hard to believe, but your fat cells are supposed to send satiety signals to the appetite center in your brain to turn down hunger. These signals come in the form of the hormone *leptin*—we call it "leptin the leanifier." Your fat cells release leptin to keep your brain informed about the amount of fat in your fat cells: *Plenty of fat in here, don't need to store any more. Better stop eating.* Or *Getting low in here, we need to stock up. Go eat something.*

When you're carrying too much weight, however, this hormonal messenger doesn't always function properly. Obesity is associated with *leptin resistance*, a condition in which your fat cells produce more than enough leptin, but your brain either no longer gets the cues to stop eating or refuses to accept the incoming messages as if they were "spam." This often indicates a problem with the leptin receptors in your brain. (Receptors are molecules located on the surface of cells that receive incoming chemical signals from hormonal messengers.) Sometimes, receptors lose their sensitivity and no longer recognize the messengers or their signals.

When leptin was first discovered, the scientific community thought it had found a "miracle hormone" that could cure obesity. Because leptin was associated with satiety, researchers initially thought that increasing leptin in the body would increase satiety. But additional scientific studies made us question this strategy. Newer evidence showed that obese people secrete far more leptin than lean people, which revealed that the problem wasn't with the quantity of leptin but rather with the sensitivity of the leptin receptors. In obese people, the leptin receptors had become less sensitive to the hormone.

Scientists are still debating which comes first: obesity or leptin resistance? Regardless of the answer, the two feed off each other to create a vicious cycle of weight gain. High-calorie, high-fat and high-fructose diets are associated with leptin resistance. You should also know that consuming just two out-of-control meals in a 48-hour period are enough to trigger the process that leads to leptin resistance.

Reversing leptin resistance takes more time. With Lean for Life's protein-based, low-calorie, low-fat, low-glycemic eating plan, you can begin to increase leptin sensitivity to enhance feelings of satiety.

DAY 9: MENU DAY

BECOME A MITOCHONDRIAC

What if we told you that doctors were going to start prescribing a surefire drug that would spark fat burning so you could lose more weight and keep it off for good? And what if we told you that in addition to helping you lose weight faster, this drug's "side effects" included:

- Increased energy and stamina.
- Reduced cravings.
- Burning more calories while doing *nothing at all.*
- Better moods.
- Reduced stress.
- Improved sleep.
- A younger appearance.
- Enhanced memory.
- Fewer colds and flu.
- Lower blood pressure.

With a list of benefits like this, you—and millions of other people—would be lining up to get a prescription from you doctor. We've got news for you. This "drug" already exists. It's called physical activity, and getting more of it can help you enjoy more of the benefits on this list.

One of the reasons why physical activity is so beneficial is because it increases *mitochondria.* Mitochondria are the tiny, egg-shaped structures *inside* your cells that serve as fat-burning furnaces. Too small to be seen with an ordinary microscope, there are trillions in every human body. The more mitochondrial surface you have in your cells, the easier it is for your body to burn stored fat for fuel. If you want to burn more body fat so you can shrink your fat cells, you need to increase the mitochondrial surface in your cells. How can you do this? By increasing your physical activity on a daily basis, you will increase the mitochondria in your cells. The result? It'll be easier for your body to burn stored fat for fuel and shrink your fat cells, a process you can see in "How Physical Activity Affects Fat Cells."

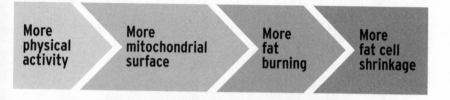

HOW PHYSICAL ACTIVITY AFFECTS FAT CELLS

Physical activity sparks a physiological process that helps you shrink fat cells.

One way we help our patients focus on this important weight-loss strategy is by helping them *visualize* mitochondria, even though they're too small to see. We created a silly mascot named "Mr. Mito" to remind our patients that *movement* matters—even the smallest movement. Think of Mr. Mito as your exercise and activity coach. He'll have plenty of tips to share with you throughout the book.

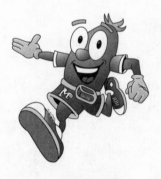

MR. MITO

Meet Mr. Mito, our mitochondria mascot.

The Inside Story from Dr. Allouche

MOVE MORE FOR MR. MITO

For just a moment, think of your body as a factory that's in the business of fat-burning. On the front lines are Mr. Mito and his crew of hard-working mitochondria. They are so valuable to your fat-burning business that Mr. Mito is your Employee of the Month every month. Because he is your factory's most prized employee, you need to treat him and his team well. If you provide them with ideal working conditions—a cool temperature and reasonable quotas are all they ask—they'll do a great job. But if the work environment is less than optimal, they'll start to slack off and might even go on strike, bringing fat burning to a screeching halt.

Now imagine that you had to work in sweltering 100-degree heat inside a factory with no air conditioning, no ventilation and no windows. And on top of that, your workload just doubled, and your boss is screaming, "Work harder!" It sounds stressful, doesn't it? You would probably be exhausted and ready to call it quits. Unfortunately, if you've been overweight or obese for a long time, this is the sort of working environment you've created for Mr. Mito and his team, and they don't like it.

More fat means Mr. Mito's department has to work harder than they need to. The fact that excess fat is associated with an increase in inflammation makes things worse. Inflammation triggers the release of chemicals called heat shock proteins (HSP) that attempt to protect Mr. Mito and his staff, but these chemicals can be, in fact, over-protective and may prevent them from doing their jobs properly. Over time, your stressed-out workers simply can't keep up with the demand, and they go on strike. That results in more fat, more inflammation and even worse working conditions for your already overworked mitochondria.

How do you get Mr. Mito and his crew up and running again? One of the best ways is to do more physical activity, which effectively increases the number of Mr. Mito's workers and lessens the workload for each one. If you have a hard time getting pumped up for physical activity, remember this: you're not just doing it for yourself, you're also doing it for Mr. Mito. He deserves it, doesn't he?

MR. MITO'S MODERATE EXERCISE PRESCRIPTION

Remember, on this program, one of the key goals is simply to "move more," so we aren't going to force you to follow a rigid fitness regimen. The majority of our patients find it easiest to start with walking as their main form of exercise. We encourage you to walk for about 30 minutes a day, five days a week—yes, it's that simple. We also want you to aim for 10,000 steps total throughout your day. This includes not only the steps you take while actively exercising, but also the steps you take while vacuuming the house, going from your office to the conference room or going from your car to your front door. If you haven't been very active, it may take time to work up to 10,000 steps. That's okay. Just do it gradually, adding about 500 steps per week. An easy way to monitor the number of steps you take on a daily basis is to wear a pedometer, accelerometer or other activity monitor. Just clip it on your belt, waistband or shoe every morning, and record the number of steps you take on your DAP.

WHEN LESS IS MORE

On this program, it's best to keep exercise in the moderate zone. Forget the "no pain, no gain" approach to exercise. You don't have to feel nauseated to know you're working out hard enough. Doctors, health researchers and fitness experts now know that a consistent program of moderate-intensity exercise can increase mitochondria, burn fat and maintain good health.

In fact, a 2013 study comparing the health benefits of walking versus running revealed—*surprise!*—walking is just as beneficial as running in reducing the risk for type 2 diabetes, high blood pressure and high cholesterol. For this study, researchers analyzed 33,060 runners and 15,045 walkers and assessed their efforts by distance rather than by time. This means they compared running three miles at a vigorous pace with walking briskly for three miles, rather than comparing running for half an hour with walking for half an hour. The takeaway here is that you can stick to walking and still get all the benefits of running, but you've got to go the distance.

More evidence on the benefits of moderate exercise comes from a 2011 trial that examined the exercise habits of 416,175 adults over a 13-year period. Compared to inactive people, those who did an average of 15 minutes daily of moderate-intensity activity—like walking, gentle jogging or cycling—increased their life span by about three years and decreased the risk of mortality from all causes by about 14 percent. Every additional 15 minutes of daily moderate-intensity exercise beyond the minimum amount of 15 minutes further reduced the risk of mortality from all causes by 4 percent.

How can you tell if you're exercising at a light, moderate or high intensity? Research from the University of New Hampshire has recently confirmed that a commonly used self-test, known as the Talk Test, is an effective tool for gauging exercise intensity.

- **Light intensity:** means that you can carry on a conversation or sing while exercising.

- **Moderate intensity:** means that you can carry on a light conversation but can't sing while exercising.

- **High intensity:** means that you can speak only in short phrases while you exercise.

If, while exercising, you can't talk without feeling short of breath, take it down a notch: your activity is not moderate enough.

After reading today's advice, are you starting to feel as though exercising enough to create mitochondria may not be as hard as you think? In addition to being easier to do and less likely to cause injury than vigorous exercise, moderate exercise has been proven to be one of the most effective ways to increase mitochondria. But moderate exercise isn't the only type of physical activity that provides these benefits. Throughout this book, you will discover a variety of types of activity that burn calories, increase mitochondria and promote fat burning to help shrink your fat cells.

FINDING THE TIME TO MOVE

Think you don't have enough time to exercise? In 2011, Japanese researchers published the results of a study that compared a single 30-minute bout of moderate exercise with three 10-minute bouts at the same intensity. And guess what they discovered? Exercising in 10-minute spurts burned *more fat* than exercising for 30 minutes continuously. This means that instead of trying to carve out a big chunk of time in your day for exercise, you can squeeze it in 10 minutes at a time. How easy is that?

Everyone—yes, even you and I—can find ways to add more activity into our daily life. In our clinics, we meet with thousands of patients each year, and when many of them hear the words *exercise* or *physical activity*, they immediately think or even say, "I hate exercise" or "I don't have the time for physical activity." As you now know, these are thought bombs planted by your inner sabotage agents in an attempt to keep you stuck in your old ways. Let me introduce you to two of our patients who had a lot of these thought bombs.

- **Stephanie, age 33, lost 18 pounds.** With a full-time job and three-year-old twins, Stephanie said she would never be able to find the time to go to the gym. That's when we told Stephanie about the Japanese study showing that just 10 minutes of activity three times a day burned more fat than exercising 30 minutes continuously. Encouraged, Stephanie looked at her daily schedule to see if there were any pockets of time where she could squeeze in 10 minutes of activity. She started taking a 10-minute walk during her lunch hour, walking her kids to the park on weekends and walking the dog for 10 minutes after dinner. Seeing how easy it was to fit in the 10-minute bouts of activity throughout her day, Stephanie said, "I can do this!"

- **Jordan, age 40, lost 35 pounds.** When Jordan first came to our clinic soon after turning 40, he was enthusiastic about trying to change his eating habits to lose the 35 pounds he had put on since he landed a high-pressure job five years earlier. But when we talked to him about the importance of moving more, he held up the palm of his hand and announced, "I hate exercise. I'm never going to do it."

As the conversation progressed, it came out that Jordan loved hiking on his local trails, which is a wonderful form of exercise. But Jordan had never equated hiking with "exercise" because in his mind, "exercise" only meant going to a gym, running endlessly on a treadmill and pumping heavy weights. Jordan didn't hate exercise. He hated specific activities associated with going to a gym. When we pointed out to Jordan that hiking *is* exercising, he was thrilled, and it changed his entire mindset about his ability to succeed on the program.

Take a few moments and consider the way you think about exercise. Do you have any inner sabotage agents trying to prevent you from engaging in physical activity? Practice thought control to silence those inner saboteurs so you can start moving more and enjoying it.

DAY 10: MENU DAY

LEARN TO MANAGE STRESS AND YOU'LL LEARN TO MANAGE FOOD

Traffic. Screaming children. Deadlines. Financial struggles. Fighting with your spouse. Caring for an ailing parent. Knee pain. Health problems. Weight issues. Argh! Life is stressful and getting more stressful by the minute. Trying to juggle your job, your family and your finances, in addition to an overwhelming flood of emails, texts, Facebook messages, Twitter feeds and more can keep you seriously stressed out. You're not alone.

According to the American Psychological Association's 2012 Stress in America survey, 39 percent of adults said that their stress had increased over the past year, and 44 percent said it had increased over the past five years. A weakened economy hasn't helped. The poll showed that 80 percent of Americans said that the economy caused them significant stress. You can expect to feel stress at various times throughout your program. You might even be feeling stressed today.

When stress hits, what do you do? If you're like many people, you probably try to soothe yourself with cookies, potato chips, pizza or ice cream (or all of the above). Yes, most people turn to exactly these things. While food indulgences may calm your nerves momentarily, these splurges are often followed by additional stress about what the repercussions of eating all that junk food might be—gaining weight, exacerbating your health problems, worsening your knee pain and the list goes on and on. So you turn to food once again for solace. And the cycle of using food as a coping strategy continues. Don't be discouraged. Throughout this program you'll learn healthy strategies to use instead.

The Inside Story from Dr. Allouche

STOP STRESSING ABOUT STRESS

We're going to let you in on a little secret: *sometimes stress can be a good thing.* Let's say you come face to face with a 500-pound grizzly bear in the woods. That's when your body's natural stress response kicks into high gear–pumping out cortisol and releasing glycogen (sugar) that is stored in your liver to give you the heightened energy you need to fight off that bear (okay, that's not very likely) or run for your life. You choose to run, and lucky for you, the bear loses interest in chasing you. But by sprinting as fast as you can, you deplete those energy supplies, and your body returns to its natural calm state so you can go back to enjoying your walk in the woods.

The problem is that in today's world, stress doesn't usually come in the form of that *very rare* meeting with a 500-pound bear. Stress assaults us nonstop on a psychological level, which means that we experience the rise in stress hormones like cortisol, but because our "predator" doesn't require us to fight or run, we never burn off those extra stores of sugar. The result is that energy is instead stored as fat. And all that extra cortisol just hangs around in our bodies promoting water retention and more fat accumulation, especially a dangerous type known as *visceral fat* that deposits itself around our organs and increases our risk for serious disease.

Because we don't *need* to fight or run, our bodies remain in a perpetual state of stress. It's as if we're at war, and our bodies are prepared to go into battle *at any moment*. Is it any wonder we all feel more on edge than ever? Being at this heightened state of readiness takes a toll on gut bacteria, too. A 2011 study from researchers at the Ohio State University shows that chronic stress leads to imbalances in gut microflora that weaken the immune system. All of these brain, body and gut changes contribute to inflammation, water retention and, ultimately, more fat, which leads to even more inflammation. Some experts say that the more stressed you are, the more you train your brain to create more stress. It's another one of those vicious circles, and trying to get it under control can be a real challenge.

That's where any form of moderate movement comes in. Without a need to fight or run, we have to find other ways to calm our body's stress response. Some people turn to medication, including antidepressants or anti-anxiety pills. But did you know that antidepressant and anti-anxiety medications are often associated with further weight gain? Even more weight leads to even more stress. Others choose to self-medicate, and for many people, the number-one self-soother is food. Food acts like a drug that provides momentary relief but that ultimately packs on more pounds and also adds to your stress.

Finding healthier ways to soothe stress is the key to breaking this vicious circle. Practicing the relaxation techniques described here and throughout the book can help you go from being a super-stresser to a more carefree, *c'est la vie* type of person.

HEALTHIER WAYS TO STRESS LESS

There are a number of healthier, more effective ways to reduce the stress in your daily life. Here are some that our patients find particularly helpful. Try them all to find which ones work best for you.

- **Get a massage.** Human touch is powerful. The Touch Research Institute at the University of Miami has conducted more than 100 studies on massage therapy and has found that it decreases stress hormones, diminishes pain and much more.

- **Try self-massage.** Who says you have to spend a lot of money to enjoy the benefits of massage? The do-it-yourself approach can provide just as much relief. A University of Miami study found that a 15-minute self-massage at work reduced stress and boosted job performance. (See the "Say 'Ahhhhh,' Self-Massage" section that follows this list for a simple technique you can use to reduce tension in mere minutes.)

- **Hug someone.** Hugging, holding hands or just sitting next to a loved one—sometimes that's all it takes to calm your nerves. Beyond massage, simple physical contact has been shown to lower blood pressure and increase production of serotonin, the so-called "happiness hormone."

- **Take a time-out.** When you're having a hectic day, take a brief "time-out" to quiet your mind and relax. Admit it: sometimes it's easy to forget that just a few minutes outdoors or even just a short walk down the hall and away from your desk can make a world of difference in how you feel.

- **Breathe deeply**. If you're feeling stressed, take a few deep, soothing breaths and consciously relax your jaw. (See the "Breathe Easy" section later in this chapter for specific recommendations.)

- **Pray or meditate.** Many people find prayer and meditation extremely helpful for stress relief. Consider building as little as 5 or 10 minutes of reflection into your day.

- **Exercise.** One of the best ways to reduce stress and improve your ability to handle stress is to exercise on a regular basis. Consider meeting Mr. Mito for a brief but brisk stretch of your legs around the block.

- **Eat more omega-3s.** It's official: omega-3 fatty acids can help reduce stress levels by about 20 percent. Research shows that omega-3s are critical for brain development and balancing your moods. Recommended proteins on this program that are abundant in omega-3s include salmon, halibut, scallops, shrimp, snapper, tofu, tuna and eggs (choose eggs that are "DHA-enriched"). Many of the convenience snacks are also a good source of omega-3s and provide an optimal balance of omega-3 and omega-6 fatty acids, which you'll read about on Day 16 in chapter 6.

- **Other stress relievers.** Take a bath, listen to music or write in your journal. If you enjoy an activity and you find that it makes you feel more calm, don't discount it—*use it* to change the way you feel about your day and yourself in the moment.

Dr. Stamper Says

THE SIX ESSENTIALS—ESSENTIAL #5: LEARN TO USE RELAXATION TECHNIQUES AND STRESS LESS.

From the earliest days of his work with overweight and obese patients, Dr. Stamper noticed that people who have difficulty managing stress tend to have difficulty losing weight and keeping it off. Dr. Stamper saw that many of his patients turned to food as a stress reliever, which sabotaged their weight loss efforts.

Dr. Stamper realized that learning to manage stress in healthier ways had to be an essential part of the program. He encouraged his patients to stop using food as a tranquilizer and to start using relaxation techniques for managing stress. When his patients learned to go with the flow and stress less, they lost weight more easily.

SAY "AHHHHH," SELF-MASSAGE

We started teaching this self-massage technique to our patients in the 1970s. It is so effective it can melt away stress and tension in a matter of minutes. It can also cure a headache. It's only fair to warn you that if you're doing this correctly, you will feel some discomfort at first. Rest assured that any discomfort is only temporary, while the results will be long lasting.

1. Reach up with both hands to the base of your skull, one hand under each ear. Feel the muscles and the bones.

2. Press firmly against the bone below the ear without loosening the pressure and move your hands gently back and forth so that you cover the entire width and length of the muscle. Hold this as tightly as you can and apply pressure continuously for at least one minute. It takes that long to begin relaxing muscle tension.

3. Continue rubbing for at least another two to four minutes. The more your rub, the better it will feel.

4. Rub from the base of your skull under your ears, down the sides of your neck and out to your shoulder blades.

5. Repeat this several times a day to prevent the tension from recurring.

6. Continue this process daily. Within four to seven days, you'll find that your neck and shoulder muscles feel less tense. Note that after the first time you do this, your neck and shoulders will likely feel tender and may even be bruised. This is a natural result of having worked acidic muscles so vigorously the day before. If you allow too much time to pass between rubdowns, your neck and shoulder muscles will tighten back up and you'll have to start all over again. Begin gently until it starts feeling more comfortable; then do it as vigorously as you can.

7. Give yourself a quick checkup a few times a week. Reach beneath the base of your skull and about the middle of your neck and press firmly. If you don't experience any significant tenderness, congratulations! Your neck and shoulders are tension-free. If you do locate a trigger point that hurts—and sooner or later you're bound to—massage it away.

BREATHE EASY

Deep breathing can quickly calm stress and relax your mind. Try this technique whenever you feel stressed or anxious.

1. Stop what you're doing and unbutton your pants if they are tight. Focus on being in the present moment.

2. Pay attention to your breathing. Notice if it's fast or slow, even or uneven, shallow or deep. Feel the movement of your body as you breathe.

3. Put one hand on the center of your chest and the other just below your navel. Look at your hands—watch and feel the movement in these two areas.

4. Consciously slow your breathing, and as you inhale, breathe deeply enough that your belly rises.

5. Aim for six to eight breaths per minute.

6. Do this exercise for five to 10 minutes.

DAY 11: MENU DAY

DON'T LET YOUR FAT CELLS PREVENT YOU FROM LOSING FAT

Have you ever started munching on a box of cookies, only to find that suddenly you've reached the bottom of the box—and then wonder where all the cookies went? Our patients have. Many of our patients admit to eating whole bags of potato chips while cramming for an exam, arguing with their kids or watching a really close football game. They weren't even aware of how each individual chip *tasted*. They didn't relish the *crunch texture* as they bit into each chip. It wasn't the *perfect level* of saltiness that kept them reaching into the bag. And they definitely weren't eating because they felt *hungry*. No, they simply managed to mindlessly consume many hundreds of empty calories because they were not in a *mindful* state.

The idea of "mindless eating" has been linked to over-eating and eating the wrong foods, both of which can cause you and your fat cells to blow up like balloons. (In today's "Inside Story from Dr. Allouche," you'll discover a lot more about your fat cells and how to harness their power to help you get leaner.)

According to Brian Wansink, author of *Mindless Eating—Why We Eat More Than We Think*, the average person makes about 200 food decisions every day but puts real thought into only about 10 percent of those decisions. You can put more thought into your daily food decisions by adopting more mindful eating strategies. See "Eating With Intention + Attention = Mindful Eating" for a quick definition of mindful eating.

EATING WITH INTENTION + ATTENTION = MINDFUL EATING

EATING WITH INTENTION: Planning what, when, where and how much you're going to eat.

EATING WITH ATTENTION: Being fully engaged in the process and fully aware of what, when, where, how much and why you're eating.

Adopting mindful eating strategies can help you make better choices so you can gain control of your eating habits and your weight. As an added benefit, you will also get more enjoyment out of eating. What could be better than that? To prevent mindless eating, try one of the following today:

- Decide how much you will eat before sitting at the table.
- Use smaller dishes, plates and bowls so that portions look larger.
- Ask yourself why you're eating. (Are you hungry—or just thirsty, tired, on-edge, sad, bored or lonely?)
- Use all five of your senses while eating—notice the colors of the food, the aromas, the taste, the texture and the way it sounds when you bite into it. (*Crunch!*)
- Ask yourself if you like the food.
- Eat slowly in silence.
- Put the fork down between each bite.
- Chew your food in every area of your mouth to savor all of its flavors.
- If you're with a group, try to be the last person to begin eating.
- Don't eat in front of the TV or your computer.

The Inside Story from Dr. Allouche

12 FASCINATING FACTS ABOUT YOUR FAT CELLS THAT WILL GET YOU LEAN

1. **You have about 30 billion fat cells in your body.** Even lean people with six-pack abs have billions of fat cells.

2. **Your fat cells are more than just storage units.** For years, researchers thought our fat cells did little more than act as reservoirs for fat. But new imaging techniques have provided us with a fascinating peek inside our fat cells, indicating that our fat cells work together as an active organ.

3. **Your fat cells secrete more than 100 different hormones and chemicals.** Your thyroid gland, for comparison's sake, releases only four types of hormones. If you consider how a sluggish thyroid can contribute to weight gain, imagine what sluggish fat cells can do!

4. **If you're lean, your fat cells help keep you lean.** In lean people, fat cells are typically small in size and secrete good-guy hormones and chemicals—like leptin and adiponectin—that help reduce hunger and increase insulin sensitivity. This helps keep you lean even as you eat.

5. **Your fat cells can swell up to 50 times their normal size.** The bigger your fat cells, the more harmful chemicals they secrete and the harder it is to lose weight.

6. **If you're carrying too much weight, your fat cells work to keep you fat.** When you gain weight, your fat cells expand and don't pump out as much of the beneficial hormones. Instead, they start attacking your system with hormones that thwart weight loss and help your fat cells grow even bigger.

7. **Your body can create new fat cells.** In between your fat cells are billions more immature cells. When your fat cells get so stretched out that they just can't store

any more fat, they shuttle unused carbs or fat to these nearby cells for storage, effectively transforming them into full-fledged fat cells. Now your fat cells are not only bigger, but there are also more of them! And they're bombarding you with fat-promoting hormones.

8. **Overstuffed fat cells are invaders.** Your growing army of fat cells wants to invade every nook and cranny of your body, occupying the spaces in between your internal organs and even infiltrating your muscles. The intra-abdominal fat that envelops your organs is particularly dangerous and is linked to increased risk for heart disease, stroke and other serious diseases. And the fat in your muscles impacts your metabolism and makes it hard for Mr. Mito to do his job.

9. **Your fat cells don't die.** Like those science fiction "supersoldiers" who can take a beating and still keep fighting, your fat cells are very hard to kill. And if your body creates new fat cells, you're stuck with them.

10. **Liposuction won't solve your weight problem.** Liposuction, a medical procedure that surgically removes fat from your body, doesn't change the way your fat cells function. Your remaining fat cells will continue to spew out the harmful hormones that promote weight gain.

11. **You can shrink the size of your fat cells.** While you cannot eliminate your fat cells, you can reduce their size with the help of some powerful allies:

   - **Ketosis:** When you are in ketosis, your body must turn to the fat stored in your fat cells for fuel. This forces your fat cells to release their contents and shrink in size.

   - **A low-calorie diet:** Following a low-calorie eating plan also encourages your fat cells to spill their contents to provide energy for your body.

   - **Consuming peptides:** Peptides found in proteins increase satiety to prevent overeating so you can burn fat and deflate your fat cells.

12. **Shrinking your fat cells reverses their toxic effects.** When you shrink those fat cells back down to size, you get them working *for* you instead of against you. They release less of the harmful hormones that keep you fat and start secreting more of the good hormones that help you get and stay lean. With 30 billion "soldiers" on your side, it's much easier to win the battle of the bulge.

DAY 12: MENU DAY

THE 90-SECOND FAT-BURNING BOOSTER

Welcome to another great day in your journey to becoming Lean for Life. By now, you're seeing and feeling the positive effects of eating better, moving more and stressing less—your clothes may be feeling a bit looser, your mood is getting brighter and your energy levels are going through the roof. You may be feeling so energetic that you're ready to add a little oomph to your exercise routine. In today's "Inside Story from Dr. Allouche," you'll discover the fastest way to burn more fat and shrink more fat cells.

You're also going to see how exercise does far more for you than just burn calories while you're working out. You're going to discover how it supports your heart health by increasing something called heart rate variability (HRV), which turns out to be very important to your weight-loss efforts.

WHAT'S HRV?

HRV refers to the tiny variations in the beat-by-beat rhythm of your heartbeat. Most people think that the heart beats in perfect rhythm:

ba-dum.....ba-dum.....ba-dum.....ba-dum.....ba-dum

In reality, the rhythm of a healthy heart varies from beat to beat. For example, it might sound like this:

ba-dum.....ba-dum..ba-dum....ba-dum..ba-dum

A growing body of research shows that higher levels of HRV are associated with better physical and mental health, including:

- Increased ability to adapt to the demands of physical and mental stress of all kinds—such as emotional issues, negative thoughts (like those inner sabotage agents) and exercise.

- More behavioral flexibility, meaning it's easier to change your habits.

- Improved brain processing, which translates into better decision-making, planning and problem-solving.

Gaining control of your thoughts and emotions, making better decisions, changing your habits—this is exactly what becoming Lean for Life is all about. And increasing your HRV can help you do it.

What's most exciting about these new findings is that you have the power to gain some control over your HRV. One of the best ways to do it is with BioModification, which you read about on Day 8. Since the 1970s, we've been seeing how BioMods, such as moderate exercise, help our patients lose weight. Now, thanks to this new research, we're gaining a better understanding of the many reasons *why* these techniques have been so effective, one of which is that they all have positive effects on HRV.

In other words, if you choose to be kind to your heart by exercising and practicing other BioMod techniques that increase HRV, your heart will help you become Lean for Life! See "How to Boost HRV."

There's another way to improve HRV. In response to the mounting evidence about the benefits of higher levels of HRV, an interest in HRV biofeedback training has emerged. A 2012 study from Germany shows that HRV training not only increases HRV but also *decreases* food cravings in people who suffer from strong cravings. The researchers suggest that HRV training may be beneficial for people who are trying to change their eating behaviors. If you're interested in HRV training, check out HeartMath (heartmath.org), which offers a variety of tools and techniques to boost HRV.

HOW TO BOOST HRV

PRACTICE BIOMODS THAT IMPROVE HRV

Exercise	Meditation	Relaxation techniques
Laughter	Monitoring emotions	Weight loss
Love	Positive thoughts	
Sex	Prayer	

AVOID THINGS THAT LOWER HRV

Being sedentary	Chronic stress	Emotional distress
Chronic inflammation	Eating foods that cause inflammation	Negative thinking

The Inside Story from Dr. Allouche

90-SECOND FAT-BURNING BOOSTER

Yes, moderate exercise is a great way to increase the benefits of mitochondria and promote better health, but if you put a little more heart into your exercise for just 90 seconds, your heart will help you get a lot more out of it. Exciting new research shows that adding 90-second bursts of high intensity to your moderate exercise program causes your heart muscle to release special fat-burning peptides called *atrial natriuretic peptide* (ANP) and *brain natriuretic peptide* (BNP). As it turns out, these peptides are the *best* fat-burning agents in the human body. The more ANP and BNP you can produce, the more fat you can burn and the more your fat cells will shrink—and not just *while* you're exercising. In some people, the increased fat burning can last *all day and all night long.*

All it takes is 90 seconds—that's less time than it takes to listen to your favorite song or soft-boil an egg. Here's how you do it. Walk at a moderate pace for 10 minutes then speed up to a high intensity for 90 seconds. What defines high intensity? To find your target heart rate for high-intensity activity, start with the number 220, subtract your age, then multiply by .8. Return to your moderate pace for 10 more minutes, do another 90-second burst, then do a final 10 minutes at your moderate pace. It's a good idea to take a few minutes afterward to cool down by walking slowly. Easy, *n'est-ce pas*? See the specifics in "90-Second Fat-Burning Sample Workout."

90-SECOND FAT-BURNING SAMPLE WORKOUT

Moderate exercise	10 minutes
High-intensity burst	90 seconds
Moderate exercise	10 minutes
High-intensity burst	90 seconds

90-SECOND FAT-BURNING SAMPLE WORKOUT

Moderate exercise	10 minutes
TOTAL	**33 Minutes**

Doing the 90-Second Fat-Burning Booster workout three times a week will really ramp up fat burning. Remember, it's important to start slowly and gradually work your way up to the 90-second bursts. If you're just getting used to doing moderate exercise, start with 30-second bursts. When those begin to feel comfortable, increase the bursts to 60 seconds. When 60 seconds starts to feel easy, try the 90-second bursts.

DAY 13: MENU DAY

GIVE YOUR MOOD A PICK-ME-UP TO ENCOURAGE WEIGHT LOSS

Good news: adding fun and laughter in your life can help you lose weight and keep it off. No joke! The sad truth, however, is that many people who are overweight aren't having nearly enough fun. In fact, when our patients first come to our clinics, many of them report having some symptoms of depression. You may fall into that category, too.

This doesn't really come as a surprise, considering that mountains of evidence reveal a strong connection between depression and being overweight or obese, and in particular, to belly fat. Whatever is responsible for the relationship between the two (see today's "Inside Story from Dr. Allouche" for the latest scientific findings), it appears to be a two-way street—being depressed increases the likelihood of gaining weight, and being overweight is associated with a greater risk for depression. Talk about a double whammy—it can be tough to break free from this cycle.

About 1 in 10 Americans over the age of 12 is turning to antidepressants in search of some relief from depression. But antidepressants may have unpleasant side effects. Did you know that up to 25 percent of people taking antidepressants experience weight gain? If you're taking these medications, it may be a good time to talk with your physician or mental health professional about alternative medications. Fortunately, more and more research indicates that certain everyday behaviors can be beneficial in reducing symptoms of depression, especially when combined with other forms of treatment, such as psychotherapy and medication. We use a number of BioMod strategies that can help you inject a little more "LOL" into your life. Make a point of trying one of the following mood boosters today.

LAUGH YOUR BUTT OFF, LITERALLY

Laughing exercises the muscles in your face as well as those in your core—it's almost like doing crunches, but a whole lot more fun. It stimulates the body by raising your heart rate, increasing brain alertness, aerating your lungs, oxygenating your tissues, reducing pain and boosting your immune system. When you laugh, you increase your infection-fighting antibodies and help your body get rid of virally infected cells. Laughter can also reduce stress hormones in your body for up to 24 hours. So the next time you have a chance to watch a funny movie, tell a joke or recount a funny story, go for it!

WALK OFF BLUE MOODS

When Duke University researchers studied patients with depression, they discovered that those who took a brisk walk for 30 minutes three days a week improved as much as those who took an antidepressant. What's more, six months after the conclusion of the study, 92 percent of those who were still walking reported that they no longer felt depressed at all. When asked why exercise works so well, the lead researcher credited biochemical changes in the brain as well as social support. Many of the patients also gained a sense of accomplishment. He said that since patients were sedentary before the study they didn't think they would be successful, but when they were successful, they really felt better about themselves.

SING A HAPPY SONG

Singing has been called an antidote for stress and depression. It releases endorphins to make you feel better almost instantly, and it requires deep breathing, which acts as a stress reliever. The best part is that it doesn't matter if you have a voice that would rival Christina Aguilera or if you sound like Kermit the Frog. Too shy to belt out your favorite tune? Try humming instead. It can also boost your spirits.

DANCE WITH ABANDON

Like most forms of exercise, dancing produces feel-good endorphins and gets your heart pumping. It also presents an opportunity for social bonding and provides an outlet for self-expression. And it only takes a few minutes to feel the effects. If you're having a bad day, turn on an upbeat tune and start grooving.

SHOW THOSE PEARLY WHITES

Did you know that smiling makes other people think you're smarter, kinder, more confident and better-looking? That's the finding of research conducted by Robert Zajonc, Ph.D., of Stanford University, who concluded that a simple smile can have a profound effect on the way we feel—and on how others feel about us. What's more, it can intensify our own feelings of well-being. Scientists believe that when you smile, you constrict as many as 42 muscles in your face. This constriction decreases the amount of blood flowing to your brain and thereby cools your brain. Smiling also changes the way you breathe, causing more air to flow through your nasal passages, which also cools the brain. The cooler the brain, the happier we feel. No wonder smiling feels so good!

GET SOME SUNSHINE

Sunlight entering your body through the retina of your eye will elevate your mood and increase your energy.

SAY "OM"

Meditation, visualization and relaxation techniques, prayer, contemplation and other forms of mental training are powerful ways to reduce stress and increase your sense of well-being.

BE A LOVER

We're really talking about connecting in positive and meaningful ways with other people. Every time you have an interaction that lets you know that you are esteemed, understood and valued, you are combatting depression.

The Inside Story from Dr. Allouche

THE DOPAMINE RUSH

How do laughter, smiling and other mood boosters help fight the blues and promote weight loss? They cause the brain to release *dopamine*, a neurotransmitter that produces feelings of happiness. This is important because people who are obese tend to have fewer dopamine receptors, which means they feel less pleasure and are more likely to experience depression. Reduced pleasure may also help explain why some people over-eat. Let's look at how dopamine works when two people—Dopamine Diane with healthy dopamine production and Sad Brad with reduced dopamine receptors—take a bite of cheesecake.

DOPAMINE DIANE

1. When Diane puts that forkful of cheesecake into her mouth, she thinks, *That's decadent,* and then, *Boy, that's good.* She savors the texture on her tongue, detects a hint of lemon, and lets it slowly melt in her mouth, loving every second of it.

2. In response, the part of her brain called the nucleus accumbens releases dopamine, which makes her feel great.

3. Completely satisfied with the experience, she puts down her fork and lets her dinner companions finish off the slice.

SAD BRAD

1. When Brad bites down on a forkful of cheesecake, he barely tastes it.

2. His nucleus accumbens doesn't register the flavors and releases only a tiny hint of dopamine.

3. Without getting adequate satisfaction, Brad takes another bite, then another and then another, still seeking that dopamine hit.

4. By the time he's polished off the 900-calorie slice of cheesecake, he still hasn't gotten the feel-good payoff that Diane got from one single bite. For Brad, one bite just isn't enough.

Brad is in desperate need of a dopamine do-over. By engaging in mood boosters that can give him brief surges of dopamine throughout his day, he may be able to alleviate some of his depressive symptoms and facilitate weight loss. In turn, losing weight may further reduce depression and help put Brad on the path to becoming more like Diane.

PUT A LITTLE MORE HAPPINESS ON YOUR PLATE

Eating the Lean for Life way can naturally elevate your mood and fend off depressive symptoms. Some of the mood boosting foods you're consuming on this program include:

- **Protein:** Meat, poultry, soy, eggs and dairy are high in amino acids, which stimulate dopamine production.

- **Omega-3 fatty acids:** Cold-water fish, eggs and tofu are good sources of omega-3 fatty acids, which have been shown to reduce depression.

- **Green leafy vegetables:** Spinach, broccoli, collard greens and other greens are high in folate, which helps produce dopamine.

- **Fruits:** Bananas and oranges contain *tyrosine*, a building block for dopamine.

THAT DEPRESSING GUT FEELING

Did you know there's a link between depression and your gut? By now, you've already seen that your gut and brain communicate to regulate–or *deregulate*–appetite and satiety. You've also seen that your gut is responsible for producing the majority of your body's happiness hormone, serotonin. Newer research is increasingly finding that imbalances in gut bacteria, as well as leaky gut syndrome, are linked with depression, stress and anxiety. As you saw in chapter 1, leaky gut occurs when the contents of the gut permeate the intestinal wall, causing a system-wide inflammatory response. Some experts are suggesting that anyone with depression should be checked for leaky gut and treated if necessary.

Other researchers are investigating whether balancing gut bacteria may lessen symptoms of mood and stress disorders. In one promising study, mice were fed foods containing *lactobacillus rhamnosus*, a strain of good bacteria found in the human gut.

Compared to mice that didn't consume the beneficial bacteria, the mice that ate the bacteria exhibited significantly less behavior linked with depression, anxiety and stress.

Note that these findings resulted from animal studies and have not been performed on humans. If you've been diagnosed with clinical depression or a mood disorder or are taking antidepressants or other medication, consult your mental healthcare professional before making any changes to your treatment.

DAY 14: MENU DAY

YOUR INNER SABOTEUR: RATIONALIZATION

As Sarah headed out the front door after dinner, she chirped, "Going for my evening walk." A short while after she left, the home phone rang, and her husband, Jason, answered. It was the hospital calling, saying that Sarah's mom had fallen and broken her hip. Jason rushed out the door to try to catch up with Sarah, and when he did, he finally understood why she was having so much trouble losing weight on her weight-loss program. Rather than taking her "evening walk," Sarah was sitting in the neighborhood coffee shop, munching on a huge muffin.

Sarah immediately went into emergency rationalization mode: "What? My knee felt sore, so I figured I'd better skip my walk. And besides I hardly had anything for dinner, and the muffin is fat-free so it isn't that bad."

Sarah's ability to make excuses for her behavior is hardly unique. Humans are not only rational beings, but we are also *rationalizing* beings. Psychologists call this sort of rationalization *cognitive dissonance*; we call it a defensive barrier. As you've seen in this book, defensive barriers come to our rescue whenever we want or need to protect ourselves from unpleasant feelings, difficult situations or painful truths. Rationalizations are excuses our minds make to help explain behaviors that prevent us from reaching our goals.

People who have weight problems tend to be masterful rationalizers. How else do you explain the fact that even though being overweight increases the risk for type 2 diabetes, heart disease, and high blood pressure, people continue to over-eat and over-indulge in foods that promote weight gain and disease? The same people who say they would *never* smoke cigarettes because they're bad for your health can easily put away six slices of pizza and a pitcher of soda.

And people who are actively trying to lose weight can come up with all kinds of creative excuses to justify their behavior when they stray from their weight-loss plans.

At our clinics, we've heard every excuse you can imagine. We've also found that the two-week mark is the time when some patients are so thrilled with their results thus far that they may start feeling over-confident. They're doing so well that they begin thinking it's okay to stray from the menu plans. This is when we start hearing some of the following excuses from our patients:

- "I've been so good on my program that one fast-food meal isn't going to hurt."

- "I've lost 9 pounds already. I deserve a reward."

- "I've got this weight thing under control. I don't need to be on a program anymore."

You may be feeling this way, too. If you are, be aware that going off the menu plan at any point during this phase of the program can knock you out of ketosis and may lead to rapid weight regain. To prevent rebound weight gain, it's important to recognize that you're rationalizing. As you've already seen, rationalization, which is a defense barrier, is so detrimental to your progress that Dr. Stamper made "Learn to recognize and eliminate your defensive barriers" one of the Six Essentials of this program. The following success strategies can help you learn to recognize and eliminate defensive barriers.

1. **Accept that your defensive barriers exist.** Being in denial about rationalization will prevent you from reaching your weight-loss goals. Accepting that you may be tempted to use rationalization and denial as you progress through your program is the critical first step in eliminating them.

2. **Understand the damage that defensive barriers have created for you and replace them with healthier patterns.** Look at your past weight-loss experiences to become more aware of how you've used rationalizations and denial to justify over-eating. Can you think of one example of each? What influence did they have on your behavior? Did they really protect you, or did they harm you? Knowing what you know now, what could you have done to neutralize their power?

3. **Exercise thought control.** As you saw on Day 6 in chapter 4, thought control is a process in which you consciously recognize a negative or unproductive thought and immediately replace it with a positive, productive one. If you're thinking, *It's okay if I eat a hot-fudge sundae because I got a promotion, and I deserve to celebrate*, substitute that thought with a conscious statement, such as, *My ultimate goal is to become Lean for Life, and every day, I need to make conscious choices in order to achieve my goal. So before acting impulsively, I need to STOP and ask myself if eating a hot fudge sundae is going to help me reach my goal.* The process of thought control reminds you that your actions have consequences. By exercising thought control often enough, you can change your thoughts and feelings into patterns that will help rather than hinder you. See Day 6 for thought control exercises, and make it a habit to practice them every day.

4. **Understand that disarming defensive barriers is a process.** Even after you fully understand how rationalizations and denial get in your way, there are still going to be times when your resistance may be down and they'll get the best of you. When this happens, acknowledge that you've slipped, learn what you can from the experience and accept that you made a choice that you wouldn't necessarily make again. Sometimes, the lessons we learn from our mistakes are well worth the price we pay.

5. **Remember that there may be a part of you that still resists change.** The familiar is comforting even when it is self-defeating. It can be challenging to do things differently, even when we realize that what we've done in the past doesn't work.

6. **Be conscious of the "Not Me" Syndrome.** As you proceed with your program, pay careful attention to your thoughts and actions. Don't skip over certain days in the program because you think, *I never do that! That doesn't apply to me.* Keep an open mind and try to incorporate each day's advice into your life. You may find that your defensive barriers have been keeping you from the truth.

The Inside Story from Dr. Allouche

KEEP MONITORING YOUR PROGRESS

Research shows that self-monitoring is an important ongoing strategy for maintaining weight loss. By making it a habit to do weekly progress reports now, you will be more likely to continue doing them after you reach your goal weight. Remember, the habits you are adopting now are the habits that will help keep you Lean for Life. Fill out your "Weekly Progress Report" in Appendix F.

Now is also a good time to retake the "Quiz: What's Your PSQ (Personal Satisfaction Quotient)?" that you took in chapter 3. Has your overall satisfaction changed? If so, what changes does today's score reflect? This is also a good opportunity to review the past two weeks' DAPs. Are there any changes you want to incorporate in your program as you move into Rapid Weight Loss Week 3? More activity? Fewer snacks? More fluids? Less rationalization? The fine-tuning you do now can have an impact on your results later. Jot down the changes and improvements you can make to enhance your results in the coming weeks.'

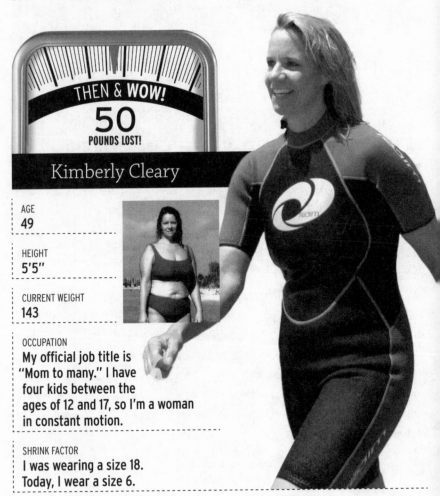

THEN & WOW!

50
POUNDS LOST!

Kimberly Cleary

AGE
49

HEIGHT
5'5"

CURRENT WEIGHT
143

OCCUPATION
My official job title is "Mom to many." I have four kids between the ages of 12 and 17, so I'm a woman in constant motion.

SHRINK FACTOR
I was wearing a size 18. Today, I wear a size 6.

I wasn't very active before I lost weight. I played an occasional game of tennis or round of golf. The idea of competing in Ironman triathlons never crossed my mind—but life is full of surprises. People tell me I seem like a different person these days, and they're right. I feel like a different person—and I really like her!

WEIGHT LOSS: I lost 50 pounds in five months—and I've kept it off for five years! I will be Lean for Life for the rest of my life.

MY "AHA MOMENT": Back when I was at my heaviest weight, I showed a new skirt to my mom and said, "Isn't this a cute little skirt?" She said, "There's nothing *little* about that skirt!" Ouch!

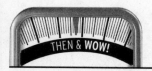

HUNGRY FOR A CHANGE: Before I lost weight, I had been dieting since I was seven years old. I tried every program and every magazine diet known to man. When I started the Lean for Life program, I was at the end of my rope. But I was also ready to give it 100 percent because it just made sense to me, and I had a feeling it would work. It was easy to follow, and I was never, ever hungry.

MOVING MORE: Once I started losing weight, I realized how much I enjoyed physical activity. I started training for an Ironman Triathlon in China, which at first seemed like an impossible goal. But I did it! When I crossed the finish line in 15 hours and 28 minutes, I was euphoric. I finished sixth in my age category. It was the most phenomenal feeling. I've since completed two more—one in Mexico and another in Texas—and I'm in training for another in Lake Tahoe. When I think of everything I've accomplished since I've lost weight, I'm totally amazed.

DO SOMETHING, DO ANYTHING: When it comes to exercise, I believe it doesn't matter *what* you do as long as you do *something*. The secret is finding something you love doing and doing it consistently.

BREATHING EASY: My asthma has improved so much since I lost weight. It feels like a weight has been literally lifted off me, which I guess is what happened. I used to have to use my inhaler a couple of times a day. These days, I can go a year without needing it.

6 RAPID WEIGHT LOSS WEEK 3:

GET LEANER AND HEALTHIER, INSIDE AND OUT

Good work! You've already completed two full weeks and are on your way to becoming Lean for Life. Our research shows that after just two weeks on this program, health conditions that stymie weight loss, such as insulin resistance and chronic inflammation, can begin to be reversed. How cool is that? We've also discovered that now is the time when our patients are more able to go beyond the nitty-gritty details of what to "do" on the Lean for Life program and start exploring what's happening inside the body—how it had been working against you to prevent weight loss and how the new habits you're developing are helping it work *for* you.

That's why this week, we'll be switching the focus to the inner body and how you're getting healthier, inside and out. Each day will begin with "The Inside Story from Dr. Allouche" and then offer practical tips and solutions to maximize your health and well-being while losing weight. This will help you zoom through Week 3 and toward your ultimate weight-loss goal. Keep up the good work!

DAY 15: PROTEIN DAY

RESIST INSULIN RESISTANCE

In our clinics, we take a medical history and do a physical exam along with a variety of lab tests on our patients to gauge their health status and determine if certain medical issues could be contributing to their weight problems. One of the most common medical conditions we detect among our patients is insulin resistance, which we've already touched on throughout this book. As a brief reminder, insulin resistance is associated with an increased risk for type 2 diabetes and promotes fat storage. Today, we'll give you the inside story on how this condition develops and what you can do—and what you're *already* doing—to reverse it.

The Inside Story from Dr. Allouche

ARE YOU ON THE FAST TRACK TO INSULIN RESISTANCE?

If you want to understand how insulin resistance occurs in the body, all you have to do is take a trip down into the busy Paris subway, the Métro. When the Métro is running smoothly, the train glides into the station, its doors peel open and the commuters on the platform swiftly enter the train. But during rush hour, the train can become so jam-packed with people that when the doors open at the station, there's no room for anyone else to squeeze in, and many irritated travelers are left stranded and waiting on the platform.

At each station, it's the same scenario—crowds try to elbow their way in but get pushed back. Now, imagine if the frustration were to boil over at a station and a near riot breaks out. The train's conductor fears another scuffle and at the next station, he refuses to open the doors. The angry mob has absolutely no chance of getting into the train. After a number of failed attempts, the riotous crowd streams back out onto the streets of Paris, desperate for alternative modes of transportation. Meanwhile, the commuters on the train are stuck and can't get off at their stop.

YOUR FAT CELLS BEHAVE A BIT LIKE THOSE MÉTRO TRAINS

Instead of having people as passengers, your fat cells store excess sugar as fat. Insulin is what escorts all that excess sugar to your fat cells, politely waiting for your fat cells to swing open their doors and then ushering the cargo inside. The same way those Métro trains can get packed to the gills with people, *some* of your fat cells can become overstuffed. When they can't handle any more incoming deposits, they try to create new fat cells to handle the extra load. But for genetic reasons, some people reach a point when they can no longer create new fat cells. That's when the overloaded, ready-to-burst fat cells send a signal to the brain, which is your body's conductor: *Maximum occupancy exceeded!*

Your brain is determined to store that fat, so it sends out more insulin in an attempt to strong-arm your fat cells into opening their doors. Your fat cells comply, but it's so crowded inside that the insulin can't get in with its cargo to be stored.

THE FINAL STRAW

Your brain keeps trying to get your fat cells to cooperate. But then one random day, you choose to chow down on something fattening. Insulin production soars in response and tries to stuff the molecular remnants of your meal into your fat cells. The doors are open, but nothing can get in. Failure.

Finally, your conductor—your brain—realizes that the situation is hopeless and instructs your fat cells to stop opening the door, which leaves insulin floating aimlessly in your body. In essence, it is at this moment that your brain *decides* that you are going to become insulin resistant. From that moment on—unless you change your eating habits—no matter how much insulin is produced, it can no longer efficiently perform its primary functions.

To make sure that insulin can't force its way in, some of your fat cells—especially those in the abdomen—begin reinforcing their walls with a form of fibrosis called *crown-like structures.* When this occurs, insulin can't open the fat cells, and the contents of these particular fat cells can't get out. This explains one of the reasons why it's so hard to lose belly fat when you have insulin resistance. Some of the fat cells have gone into lock-down mode.

What happens to all that excess sugar that the insulin was going to place in your fat cells? It now has to find a home somewhere else, so it heads to your liver, where it settles in. With time, you may develop a fatty liver, which only worsens your body's fat-burning conditions (more on this and how to combat it on Day 18).

This scenario illustrates why it's so important to intervene quickly when you first start gaining weight. By taking action early, you can avoid these issues. Rest assured, however, that even if you've already developed insulin resistance, you can still retrain your body to unlock your fat cells so they will start cooperating again. Being in ketosis is the key.

THE KETOSIS SOLUTION

By reducing carbs and being in ketosis with this program, you can outsmart your fat cells, preventing crown-like structures from developing and breaking down any crown-like structures that may have already developed. Through ketosis, you are re-training locked-down fat cells to open their doors and liberate their contents. In fact, it can take just two weeks on this program for fat cells with crown-like structures to start to remember how to release fat.

It's important to understand that while these particular fat cells may take some time to relearn how to release their contents, other fat cells in your body start shrinking as soon as you are in ketosis. The fat cells that typically respond most quickly are found in *subcutaneous fat*, which is located directly under the skin. This is the fat that you can pinch on your belly, hips and thighs, and it is what is used to measure body fat. So even while some fat cells with crown-like structures are still in the process of relearning how to release their contents, you can still be reducing your overall body fat and looking leaner.

- -

THE SIT-ITIS SYNDROME

As a society, we have developed a serious case of "sit-itis," meaning we spend way too much time sitting on our backsides, which increases our risk for obesity, insulin resistance, type 2 diabetes and metabolic syndrome. One study from 2009 that appeared in the journal *Diabetes* came to the shocking conclusion that the more time spent sitting—regardless of the amount of time spent doing moderate or vigorous activities—the higher the levels of fasting insulin, an indicator of insulin resistance. This means it doesn't matter if you spend an hour sweating it out at the gym: if you spend the rest of the day in your chair at your desk or on the couch, you're at increased risk for insulin problems.

THE ANTIDOTE FOR "SIT-ITIS"

Up-to-the-minute science is showing that moving more by using *any form of movement*—including everyday activities like housework and even fidgeting—lowers the risk. We call this incidental movement Non-Exercise Activity Thermogenesis (NEAT), and today we will show you how to maximize the weight-loss potential associated with it.

First introduced in 2006 by Dr. James Levine, author of *Move a Little, Lose a Lot*, NEAT accounts for the calories you burn from nearly all the daily activities you do other than dedicated exercise or sleeping. Using the most advanced high-tech scientific gadgetry to measure activity and calorie burning, Levine has found that increasing your amount of NEAT can help you burn an extra 500 to 1,000 calories a day. He also says that by simply converting sedentary TV time to active time, you could lose 50 pounds a year.

As you might suspect, Levine's research shows that obese people tend to perform far less NEAT than lean folks. His recommendation to people trying to lose weight is to increase NEAT throughout the day. That's a suggestion that echoes one of the essential components of the Lean for Life mantra: "move more." It is yet another example of modern-day science validating the program Dr. Stamper developed more than 40 years ago and revealing the physiological reasons behind its success. Check the list of "'NEAT' Activities That Help You Move More."

New scientific evidence is showing that moving more with NEAT lowers your risk for insulin resistance, type 2 diabetes and metabolic syndrome. In fact, a team of Australian researchers found that doing nothing more than taking extra breaks from sitting resulted in a smaller waist size, reduced BMI, and lower triglycerides and blood sugar levels following a meal. It's important to point out that the participants in this study made absolutely *no changes to their diet,* so imagine how much more of a benefit you'll get when you combine NEAT with the Lean for Life eating plan. Now that's neat!

"NEAT" ACTIVITIES THAT HELP YOU MOVE MORE

- Cooking
- Doing dumbbell curls, marching in place or stretching while watching TV
- Doing "invisible crunches" while standing in line or driving
- Fidgeting
- Folding laundry
- Gardening
- Getting dressed
- Giving your kids a bath
- Grocery shopping
- Having "walking" meetings
- Housekeeping
- Loading the dishwasher
- Lunging while vacuuming
- Mowing the lawn
- Playing with your kids
- Shoveling snow
- Squatting while sorting laundry
- Standing
- Taking the stairs
- Walking
- Walking the dog
- Walking up the escalator
- Washing the car

DAY 16: MENU DAY

COOL INFLAMMATION TO IGNITE WEIGHT LOSS

Today, you're going to discover how chronic inflammation can put the brakes on weight loss, and you'll meet the culprits, including pro-inflammatory foods, that cause it. We'll also show you how to determine if you have chronic inflammation and then introduce you to some simple eating strategies that can turn down the heat.

EAT TO COOL INFLAMMATION

To get inflammation to chill out, you just have to follow the Lean for Life recommendations for eating as well as for moving more and stressing less (more on these tomorrow). That's because on this program, you're adopting a number of eating habits that have been shown to calm inflammation.

The Inside Story from Dr. Allouche

CHRONIC INFLAMMATION—HAS IT BEEN KEEPING YOU FROM LOSING WEIGHT?

You've probably heard about inflammation in the news recently. It's been vilified as the culprit behind everything from obesity to heart disease to cancer. But inflammation isn't always a bad thing. In fact, it's part of the body's natural response to injury.

Let's say you get a splinter in your finger—ouch! The tissues in your finger send out an S.O.S. message that ignites the inflammatory response. Your body races into action to protect the area from harmful germs and begin repairing the damage. This temporarily makes your finger red, swollen and painful, but it is an essential part of the healing process. When your finger is healed, the inflammatory response is extinguished, and things go back to the status quo.

Chronic low-grade inflammation is very different. It's as if your body thinks it has been pricked by millions of tiny internal splinters. Your body's natural repair response is ignited, but it doesn't get extinguished. It continues to spread like a slow-burning fire throughout your body and even into your brain. Instead of helping you, chronic inflammation promotes a host of problems, including all those things you've probably heard about in the media: insulin resistance, type 2 diabetes, heart disease, stroke, Alzheimer's disease, obesity and cancer. It's also been linked to gut inflammation and conditions such as irritable bowel syndrome, Crohn's disease and ulcerative colitis.

WHAT'S CAUSING CHRONIC INFLAMMATION?

A POOR DIET
Pro-inflammatory foods include sugar, refined carbohydrates, trans fats, hydrogenated fats and foods high in omega-6 fatty acids (see the next section). Inadequate fiber intake also contributes to the problem. Dietary fiber nourishes the beneficial bacteria in your gut, which helps maintain the proper balance of your microflora. When you

aren't eating enough fiber, it may allow harmful bacteria to proliferate, which sparks a veritable battle of the bugs, with good bugs attempting to kill off bad bugs. You might think that destroying the bad critters would be beneficial for you, but that's not always the case. The bad bugs contain a highly inflammatory substance called *lipopolysaccharides* (LPS) that is released upon their demise. LPS irritates the intestinal wall as well as the nerve cells that line the gut, causing inflammation. Because 10 percent of your neurons are located in your gut, this irritation is reported immediately to the brain, which also experiences inflammation.

EATING TOO MANY OMEGA-6 FATTY ACIDS IN RELATION TO OMEGA-3 FATTY ACIDS

Did you know that omega-3 and omega-6 fatty acids can impact inflammation? As you've seen already, omega-3 fatty acids are found in healthy foods like salmon, tuna and watercress. Likewise, omega-6 fatty acids are found in healthy foods, such as vegetables and eggs, but they are also found in many packaged cookies, cakes, crackers and other processed foods. Your body needs omega-6s for numerous physiological functions, but the key to optimal health lies in the ratio of omega-6 to omega-3 being consumed.

Some experts suggest that humans evolved eating equal amounts of omega-3s and omega-6s. That's a far cry from what we're consuming today. In the U.S., we're gobbling up far too many omega-6s in relation to omega-3s. Experts estimate our ratio of omega-6 to omega-3 may be as high as 40 to 1, which is far greater than the 5 to 1 ratio we consumed just 100 years ago. Eating too many omega-6s in relation to omega-3s is believed to contribute to inflammation, in addition to obesity, autoimmune diseases, heart disease, depression and more.

ABDOMINAL FAT AND OBESITY

A growing body of evidence points to excess weight, and in particular to belly fat, as one of the causes of chronic inflammation. Those plumped-up fat cells around your midsection pump out molecules called *cytokines,* which emit inflammatory signals. The bigger your fat cells and the more of them there are, the more inflammation that results.

Obesity is also linked to inflammation in an area of the brain called the hypothalamus. The hypothalamus is involved in regulating appetite, and inflammation in this area disrupts the function of an important hormone called leptin. That's the satiety hormone that tells you when you're full, and if it isn't working properly, you feel hungry all the time no matter how much you eat. Inflammation in this part of the brain also impairs insulin signaling and is related to insulin resistance.

HAPPY HOUR

Research shows that heavy drinkers tend to have higher markers of inflammation, so if you're hitting the bars for happy hour on a daily basis or regularly enjoying too much wine with dinner, you could be encouraging inflammation.

INSULIN RESISTANCE

On Day 15, you learned how insulin resistance can occur when your fat cells run out of storage room. New research is showing that insulin resistance also plays a role in inflammation and that the two conditions fuel each other dangerously. The jury is still out, however, as to which one comes first—insulin resistance or inflammation.

MENOPAUSE

Changes in hormone levels associated with menopause can cause low-grade, systemic inflammation. Menopause is also linked to an increase in abdominal fat, which ramps up the secretion of cytokines and adds to chronic inflammation.

ENVIRONMENTAL IRRITANTS AND ALLERGENS

It's unfortunate, but just breathing can result in inflammation. That's because every day, we come in contact with thousands of environmental toxins—pollution in the air we breathe, pesticides in the foods we eat, toxins in the cleaning products we use and more. If your body isn't able to eliminate all these toxins effectively, it can cause your immune system to go into hyperdrive, adding to systemic inflammation.

PSYCHOLOGICAL STRESS

Unrelenting stress can trigger physical responses in the body that contribute to chronic inflammation.

LACK OF SLEEP

New research is revealing that skimping on shut-eye results in an increase in inflammation blood markers. When sleep is interrupted, the release of the stress hormone cortisol spikes and levels of glucagon rise, which can elevate blood sugar levels. These may also contribute to inflammation.

HOW DO YOU KNOW IF YOU'RE FANNING THE FLAMES OF INFLAMMATION?

Your doctor can detect inflammation with a simple blood test called C-Reactive Protein (CRP). CRP is produced by your liver, and it rises when there is inflammation in your body. The drawback of the CRP test is that although it can detect inflammation, it can't indicate exactly where the inflammation is in the body—whether it's localized in a specific area, such as an arthritic knee, or widespread throughout your body.

High levels of CRP are thought to be an indicator of increased risk for heart disease. Here's how to interpret your CRP test results, according to the American Heart Association:

> **< 1.0:** low risk for heart disease
>
> **1.0 - 3.0:** average risk for heart disease
>
> **> 3.0:** high risk for heart disease

EAT ANTI-INFLAMMATORY FOODS

Choosing foods that are known to reduce inflammation is one of the best ways to cool that inner flame. The majority of the foods you are eating on this program are considered anti-inflammatory, such as:

- Lean protein.
- Fruits—citrus fruits contain the essential antioxidants vitamin C and vitamin E.
- Dark leafy green vegetables—high in vitamin K.
- Tomatoes—contain lycopene, a potential antioxidant.
- Low-fat dairy—in one study, people who ate 3.5 dairy servings per day had lower inflammation than those who ate only half a serving.
- Whole grains—a study found that consumption of the dietary fiber in whole grains resulted in lower levels of CRP.
- Foods high in omega-3 fatty acids—these foods are indicated on the "Lean Foods" list in chapter 2.

EAT A LOW-CALORIE DIET

Reducing your calorie intake, as you are doing on this program, can cool inflammation. That's the finding from a 2012 study by researchers at the Fred Hutchinson

Cancer Research Center in Seattle, Washington. In this trial, 439 overweight or obese postmenopausal women spent one year following one of four regimens:

- Low-calorie diet.
- Aerobic exercise (225 minutes a week of moderate to vigorous activity).
- Low-calorie diet and exercise combined.
- Control (no diet or exercise).

Women in the low-calorie diet group as well as those in the group implementing the low-calorie diet plus exercise who lost more than 5 percent of their body weight reduced markers of inflammation compared to the exercise-only group and the control group that didn't diet or exercise. The bottom line? Getting leaner cools the inferno within.

LOSE WEIGHT

Losing just 2.2 pounds reduces levels of CRP, according to a review of 33 studies in the *Archives of Internal Medicine*. When you follow this program, you will shed pounds and reduce abdominal fat, both of which cool inflammation.

FLIP THE SWITCH ON YOUR OMEGA-6:3 RATIO

Research shows that omega 6:3 ratios in the neighborhood of 5 to 1 offer protection against cardiovascular disease, cancer and inflammation. To improve your ratio, increase consumption of foods high in omega-3 and reduce—but don't necessarily eliminate—foods containing omega-6.

DAY 17: MENU DAY

DON'T FAN THE FLAME

Because chronic inflammation is so detrimental to your health, we devote a second day to more tips on how to alleviate it. Controlling inflammation isn't just about eating better. If your body is under attack from inflammation, you need to relax...literally! Learning to move more and stress less with the BioModifiers you read about on Day 8 in chapter 5 can calm your nerves and, as science now shows, calm inflammation, too. New research also confirms that positive thoughts and affirmations can have a significant impact on health and can help fight chronic inflammation. Today, we reveal what else you can do to get inflammation to chill out.

The Inside Story from Dr. Allouche

STAGE A PROTEST AGAINST INFLAMMATION!

In France, it seems that people are always taking to the streets to protest something. In some cases, these popular revolts have resulted in ousting a politician from office or overturning an unpopular government policy. It's time for you to take a cue from the French and start protesting against the inflammation inside you. By taking action, you can reduce or even extinguish that flame and turn your body into a low-inflammation zone.

To take an anti-inflammation stance, you just have to follow the Lean for Life program, which encourages you to adopt habits—eat better, move more, stress less—that have been shown to calm inflammation. Yesterday, you discovered tips on eating better to reduce inflammation. Today, you'll see how moving more and stressing less can help.

MOVE MORE

Moving more is a key component of the Lean for Life program, and it is also one of the habits that scientific research says helps put the kibosh on inflammation. For example:

- Researchers at the Centers for Disease Control (CDC) analyzed data from 13,748 American adults and found that those who participated in physical activity on a regular basis had lower CRP levels than people who were sedentary.

- A year-long trial involving sedentary, overweight, or obese postmenopausal women between the ages of 50 and 75 showed that it's never too late to get moving. Women in the trial, which was published in 2009 in *Medicine & Science in Sports & Exercise*, who exercised at a moderate pace for about 45 minutes a day, five days a week, decreased their CRP levels by 10 percent.

- In 2012, a team of researchers from Canada's University of Sherbrooke enlisted 52 obese postmenopausal women aged 50 to 70 to participate in exercise training for six months. Not only did they see improvements in their body weight, waist size, lean body mass and fat mass, but they also found that their levels of the satiety hormone leptin increased while markers of inflammation decreased.

STRESS LESS

Did you know that stressing about stressful events raises levels of inflammation? In 2013, researchers from Ohio University found that ruminating on something stressful increased levels of CRP. A 2012 study appearing in the *Journal of Physiological Anthropology* linked everyday stress with an increased risk for metabolic syndrome, which is associated with inflammation. The rest of today's advice focuses on strategies to calm stress and reduce inflammation.

DEVELOP AN INNER SMILE

To help people stress less, which has been shown to reduce inflammation, Dr. Stamper encourages people to cultivate what he calls an "inner smile," which is another form of the BioMods mentioned on Day 8 in chapter 5. He counsels people who are experiencing frustration on the program to pause, take a deep breath, hold it briefly and then visualize an internal smile as they exhale. We like to tell patients to imagine their cells with smiley faces ☺. Our patients who regularly do this report an immediate change in attitude.

Did you know that a simple smile can trigger the release of hormones that make you feel happy? Or that a frown can fire off a cascade of stress hormones? Evidence is mounting that our facial expressions influence our moods, perhaps even more than our moods affect our facial expressions. Consider a study from researchers at the University of Cardiff who looked at people who received special injections of Botox designed to deaden the frown muscles. The folks who couldn't frown were happier and less anxious than people who had not received the frown-inhibiting treatment.

For decades, experts have been recommending "smile therapy" as a way to reduce stress hormones, stabilize moods, reduce pain, induce relaxation and speed healing. Maintaining an inner smile, or a true facial smile, through times of trouble or frustration can be a source of comfort that calms you and buoys your spirits.

RELAX

As previously mentioned, being able to relax your body and calm your mind has profound positive effects on your physical and mental health. It may, in fact, help reduce inflammation. Here are a few simple instructions for a basic relaxation exercise.

1. Make time—preferably 10 to 20 minutes twice a day—when you have privacy and are free of distractions. With our lives as busy as they are today, we need to "make time" since most of us rarely seem to have "extra time."

2. Sit or lie in a comfortable position.

3. Close your eyes.

4. Let go of muscle tension.

5. Gently dismiss your thoughts and mental distractions by letting them float on by without becoming involved with them. Some people find it helpful to focus on a word or short phrase to repeat during this exercise, such as *one*, *peace* or *love*.

6. Become aware of your breathing, and continue to breathe naturally as you repeat your focus word when you exhale.

7. After 10 to 20 minutes, return to your surroundings by sitting quietly for a couple of minutes before slowly opening your eyes.

PRAY

In his research over the past 30 years, Herbert Benson, M.D., the father of the "relaxation response," has discovered that prayer reduces stress, which helps fight inflammation, and promotes feelings of peace and tranquility in those who practice it. Larry Dossey, M.D., former chief of staff at Humana Medical Center in Dallas, came to the same conclusion. In his review of more than 130 research studies, he concluded that prayer helps people overcome and prevent headaches, anxiety, high blood pressure and heart attacks. One study conducted by the National Institute for Health Care Research showed that Canadian college students with strong religious ties were better able to handle stress and had higher positive feelings than other students.

MEDITATE

Meditation, as previously mentioned, is a proven stress reliever that calms frayed nerves. Now, thanks to a 2013 study published in *Brain, Behavior, and Immunity*, we're learning that forms of meditation or mindfulness may also play a role in reducing chronic inflammation. But who says you have to sit cross-legged and burn incense to meditate? In the Buddhist tradition, there are many different ways to meditate. One of the easiest to learn is the walking meditation. It's like taking a walk, but with heightened awareness of your surroundings. You slow your pace and open your heart to the sights and sounds along the path.

Thich Nhat Hanh, a Buddhist monk and Nobel Peace Prize nominee, has written about the joys of this simple practice. Here is a quote from his book, *The Long Road Turns to Joy:*

> *Walking meditation is meditation while walking. We walk slowly, in a relaxed way, keeping a light smile on our lips. When we practice this way, we feel deeply at ease, and our steps are those of the most secure person on Earth. All our sorrows and anxieties drop away, and peace and joy fill our hearts. Anyone can do it. It takes only a little time, a little mindfulness, and the wish to be happy.*

Walking can be done in so many different ways. In this, and in everything else, you have choices: power walking or meditation walking? Every day, the choice is yours.

USE AFFIRMATIONS

On Day 8 in chapter 5, you learned that your thoughts are powerful. But did you know that they are strong enough to fight inflammation? In several studies published in the *Archives of Internal Medicine* in 2012, researchers found that patients who used positive health affirmations were more likely to engage in healthy lifestyle behaviors. And as you've seen, adopting healthy lifestyle behaviors is the key to a whole new you. The science is clear: Affirmations, as previously mentioned in chapters 2 and 4, are a healthy habit to get into. Affirmations are positive personal statements that you create, write down and then repeat to yourself over and over. Effective affirmations highlight the following:

- **Positive behavior:** State what you are doing rather than what you are *not* doing. Example: *I enjoy eating healthy foods that nourish my body* rather than *I am not eating junk food anymore.*

- **Positive feelings:** Describe what you want rather than what you do *not* want. Example: *I am becoming healthy, strong and lean* rather than *I don't want to be fat anymore.*

- **Positive commitment:** Focus on firm statements written in the present tense rather than tentative or future statements. Example: *I am succeeding at becoming Lean for Life* rather than *I hope to become Lean for Life.*

At first, the notion of being able to enhance your self-confidence by making positive statements about yourself may sound like New Age psychobabble. But while the "power of positive thinking" may be a cliché, the fact is positive thinking has a positively powerful impact on your health. Even if you feel uncomfortable making statements you think or feel aren't "true" right now, do it anyway. See the results for yourself.

WHEN TO DO AFFIRMATIONS

Many of our patients recite an affirmation before they get out of bed in the morning and in the evening as they prepare to fall asleep. That way, the affirmation is the first and last message they hear each day. These are the times when you're most likely to be in a relaxed, receptive state of mind. In order for the affirmation to become a routine part of your thinking, it's necessary to experience it in a deeper, more "whole body" kind of way rather than merely on a "thinking" level.

An affirmation that comes from your heart will always be appropriate for you, even when you're asserting something that doesn't quite feel real yet. If you deliver the message to yourself often enough, it will begin to feel real. And that's the point. You make a choice as to how you want to be and then help yourself become that person. Go ahead and try it.

CREATING YOUR AFFIRMATIONS

As you create your affirmations, remember that they are always personal "I" statements. That's because they're about you and no one else. Also be sure that your affirmations are in the present tense. Say "I am..." rather than "I will..." and you will come from a position of having already achieved your stated desire.

Now that you have an understanding of affirmations and how you can benefit from using them, it's your turn to come up with some you can use. These sample affirmations may spark some ideas:

I have everything I need to be healthy.

The food I'm eating makes me healthy and lean.

I feel wonderful when I exercise.

I am filled with energy.

I am a problem solver.

I can handle whatever challenges life gives me.

I am proud of myself for being a patient, kind person.

I am enjoying becoming Lean for Life.

I am having fun being active.

I am becoming healthy, strong and lean.

I am smiling.

I enjoy sticking with my program.

Write three affirmations on a sheet of paper. Revise them until they feel right to you. Do they highlight positive feelings? Do they encourage positive behavior? Do they affirm your positive commitment? Are they "I" statements? When your affirmations feel right, repeat them to yourself out loud and often.

DAY 18: MENU DAY

SAY *"NON, MERCI"* TO THE FOIE GRAS

Your liver is the second-largest organ in your body, and this amazing piece of internal machinery plays a role in numerous vital processes, including:

- Digesting fats, proteins and carbohydrates.
- Building proteins.
- Maintaining blood sugar levels.
- Cleansing your blood.
- Producing bile.
- Secreting enzymes that aid in fat burning.

- Storing nutrients and glycogen.
- Metabolizing hormones (thyroid).
- Metabolizing medications and alcohol.

Anything that messes with your liver can have a negative impact on other bodily processes and can make it harder for you to lose weight. Today, you'll discover what causes your liver to get fat and how you can leanify your liver so it will shrink your fat cells. In addition, just as there are "invisible" conditions inside your body that can slow your weight loss, there are ideas lurking in your brain that can derail your progress. We call these the "hidden payoffs of being overweight"—don't worry, we'll explain what this means in a moment.

The Inside Story from Dr. Allouche

SKIP THE FOIE GRAS

The French adore *foie gras,* a rich, buttery gourmet delicacy made from the enlarged liver of a duck or goose that has been specially fattened. But what you may not know is that 10 million French have *foie gras* in their own body! And as many as one in four Americans have it, too. It's called *non-alcoholic fatty liver disease* (NAFLD), and it develops when there is too much fat in the liver. In some people, the fatty liver develops inflammation and scar tissue, which is a more serious condition known as *non-alcoholic steatohepatitis* (NASH) that can permanently damage the liver and prevent it from functioning properly.

WHO IS AT RISK FOR FATTY LIVER?

As many as one in four Americans has NAFLD, and about 2 to 5 percent of adults in the United States have NASH. Chances are that if you have either type of fatty liver disease, you don't know it because there are typically no or few symptoms. Basically, if you're overweight or obese, or if you have insulin resistance or type 2 diabetes, you're at increased risk for fatty liver.

- More than 70 percent of people with NASH are obese.

- Up to 75 percent of people with NASH have type 2 diabetes.

- Almost all people with NASH have insulin resistance.

If you suspect that you might have NAFLD or NASH, ask your doctor to test your liver function.

WHAT MAKES A LEAN LIVER GET FAT?

As a general rule, anything that overtaxes your liver can contribute to a fatty liver. Some of the most common causes include the following:

- **Being overweight.** As previously mentioned, your fat cells secrete cytokines that promote inflammation, and these cytokines target the liver.

- **Not getting enough physical activity.** When you're sedentary, you're more likely to develop insulin resistance, which is associated with more fat being deposited in the liver.

- **Consuming too many trans fats and hydrogenated fats.** These harmful fats target the liver and can lead to inflammation.

- **Eating too many omega-6 fatty acids.** Consuming too many omega-6 fatty acids—found in corn, wheat germ and vegetable oils (corn, safflower, soybean, sunflower and more)—promotes inflammation and contributes to fatty liver disease.

- **Ingesting hormones in food.** About two-thirds of the cattle raised to provide beef in the United States are given hormones to promote growth. Dairy cows are also given hormones to increase milk production. These hormones overwork the liver and cause inflammation.

- **Ingesting pesticides in foods.** Pesticides mimic the effect of estrogens, which stimulate the proliferation of fat cells and the storage of fatty acids in those cells. Estrogens are metabolized by the liver and increase inflammation.

- **Gut inflammation.** Eating a diet high in saturated fats contributes to gut inflammation, which is tied to liver inflammation.

- **Drinking alcohol.** Consuming too much alcohol causes inflammation of the liver.

- **High LDL cholesterol.** High cholesterol levels have been associated with increased risk for fatty liver disease.

- **Consuming too much fructose.** A high-fructose diet contributes to insulin resistance and obesity and dysregulates liver metabolism.

THE FRUCTOSE FACTOR—A NOT-SO-SWEET STORY

Fructose is the natural sugar found in fruits and vegetables. If it's natural, then it must be good for you, right? Not always. When fructose is consumed in small amounts in whole fruits and veggies, it's okay because the fiber content in these foods helps your body metabolize it in a healthy way.

Most of us, though, aren't getting our fructose from these healthy sources. Instead, we're getting it in the form of high-fructose corn syrup (HFCS), a processed sugar which was introduced in the United States in the 1970s and has become very popular in the food industry since it is inexpensive to make and very shelf stable. HFCS can be found in sodas, packaged baked goods, ketchup, mayonnaise and many other processed foods that are devoid of dietary fiber. Just 100 years ago, the average American consumed about 15 grams daily of fructose in its natural form in fruits and veggies. Today, we're ingesting an average of 55 grams per day, mostly in the form of HFCS. Some experts estimate that 16 percent of our overall calorie intake now comes from fructose. Considering that Americans drink an average of more than 50 gallons of soda per year, it's easy to see where all those calories are coming from.

That's bad news for your waistline and your health. Research shows that consuming fructose doesn't dampen appetite and may in fact increase it, leading to overeating and being overweight. It's particularly bad for your liver because it is the *only* organ in your body that can metabolize fructose. Your liver cells struggle to break down high doses of fructose, turning it into harmful levels of fatty acids, such as triglycerides. These end up getting stored in the liver as fat.

CAN YOUR LIVER BECOME LEAN FOR LIFE, TOO?

If you have a fatty liver, you can help it get lean again. Understand that there is currently no medical cure for NAFLD or NASH, but by following the Lean for Life program, you will be doing exactly what the medical community recommends to people with these conditions:

- Lose weight.
- Eat a healthy diet.

- Increase physical activity.

- Eliminate HFCS from your diet, especially in ready-to-eat foods (read the nutrition labels!).

Just remember, a leaner liver means a leaner you, and vice versa. So love your liver and treat it with the TLC it deserves, and it will love you back.

THE HIDDEN PAYOFFS OF BEING OVERWEIGHT

When we first meet our patients, we ask them a surprising question: "What are the benefits of being overweight?" They usually look at us as if we have a hole in our head before saying, "None." When we pose this same question after they've achieved a leaner physique, they often have a very different response. Take Colleen, for example, a 32-year-old entertainment attorney who lost 109 pounds on the program while gaining a healthy dose of self-awareness.

"There were benefits I wasn't even aware of until I had to give them up," she explains. "My weight was a convenient excuse for anything that wasn't working in my life. If I lost a case, for example, I would tell myself it was because the jury didn't like fat women. One day it dawned on me—my fat was taking a toll on my self-respect as well as on my body."

Several months into her program, Colleen also came face-to-face with a truth she had long denied—for 10 years she had been using her fat to insulate herself from men. "I was never comfortable with all of the attention I got from boys in high school," she admits. "The more weight I put on, the less of a problem it was. Without my realizing it, this was my way of protecting myself. At that point in my life, it never occurred to me that I could be a thin, attractive woman and not be hassled or harassed by men."

Colleen's story is more common than you might think. What have been *your* hidden payoffs for being overweight? Avoiding relationships? Making excuses for failures in your life? Keeping you chained to a job you don't like? This program is designed to help you gain awareness of the many things that could be contributing to your weight problems. By identifying your hidden payoffs, you will be taking an important step toward ensuring that you don't lapse into self-defeating patterns of behavior. (See Day 7 in chapter 4 for more on defensive barriers.)

DAY 19: MENU DAY

SLEEP IT OFF

Can you sleep your way lean? It can definitely help. Not getting enough sleep, on the other hand, can hurt your efforts to lose weight. Skimping on shut-eye has been found to increase appetite and the number of calories people consume. Typically by Day 19, we find that Lean for Lifers are ready to look at their overall lifestyle, including snoozing habits, to determine if a lack of adequate sleep has been preventing them from losing weight. Here, we'll explain how lack of sleep affects your weight and give you tips to help you get the restorative shut-eye you need.

The Inside Story from Dr. Allouche

SLEEP ON THIS

In the United States, nearly 30 percent of adults get less than six hours of sleep per night. That's troublesome, considering that scientific evidence clearly indicates that people who skimp on sleep tend to gain more weight than people who snooze for the recommended seven to eight hours a night. What's sleep got to do with the size of your thighs? A lot! Chew on this.

LACK OF SLEEP DEREGULATES APPETITE HORMONES

Did you know that your body's appetite hormones are regulated primarily while you slumber? Let's do a quick refresher course on two of these important hormones. Ghrelin, which stimulates the appetite, is like a pesky gremlin that makes your stomach growl and stimulates fat storage. Leptin, which suppresses the appetite, acts like a natural leanifier that encourages you to put down your fork and stimulates energy expenditure.

When you're trying to lose weight, there's no doubt that leptin can work for you, while ghrelin may fight you every step of the way. When you don't get enough sleep, leptin production wanes. In one study, healthy men slept for just four hours a night for two nights, then slept for 10 hours a night for an additional two nights, and researchers charted their ghrelin and leptin levels, as well as their hunger. After the restricted sleep, 18 percent of the guys experienced a drop in leptin levels, and 24 percent had higher concentrations of ghrelin. And hunger levels? They increased by 24 percent, while the appetite for fatty foods and carbohydrate-rich fare jumped by 30 percent!

These changes in appetite hormones help to explain something we've all experienced. When you don't sleep well, you feel hungrier and want to eat more junk food the next day. A growing body of research shows that people who skimp on sleep tend to snack more and consume more calories overall.

In one study from the University of Chicago, a team of researchers found that when people slept only five and a half hours per night, they didn't eat more at their main meals, but they did eat more calories from snacks and consumed more snacks with high carbohydrate content. This same team of researchers found that when you cut back on sleep, it significantly reduces the amount of fat you lose while dieting. In this study, dieters who reduced sleeping duration from eight and a half hours to five and a half hours decreased fat loss by 55 percent.

In another trial, Marie-Pierre St.-Onge, a research associate at the New York Obesity Research Center, used brain imaging to show that the sight of unhealthy food activates the brain's reward center in people with restricted sleep. When these same people viewed images of healthy foods like vegetables and fruits, the reward and cravings networks in their brains did not activate.

SKIMPING ON SLEEP BUMPS UP BLOOD SUGAR LEVELS

Not snoozing enough leads to other problems associated with weight gain, including an impairment in your body's ability to regulate blood sugar levels. As you sleep, your body releases glucagon, which causes blood sugar levels to rise. In response, your body releases insulin to lower blood sugar levels. With adequate sleep, this natural rise and fall results in blood sugar levels being at their lowest in the morning when you wake up. Research shows that when you routinely get less than six hours of sleep per night, fasting blood sugar levels increase. High fasting blood sugar levels are associated with pre-diabetes and type 2 diabetes, both of which are linked to increased risk for obesity.

INADEQUATE SLEEP CRANKS UP CORTISOL

As you've already seen, the stress hormone cortisol increases appetite and promotes belly fat and insulin resistance. When you're sleep deprived, cortisol levels increase dramatically. In one study, sleeping just four hours a night for six nights caused cortisol levels to spike, indicating a low sensitivity to insulin, which is a sign of insulin resistance.

LACK OF SLEEP CONTRIBUTES TO CHRONIC INFLAMMATION

Lack of sleep increases inflammation levels, which stalls weight loss. Data from one study showed that people who get six or fewer hours of sleep had higher levels of CRP as well as other inflammation markers. On average, CRP levels were about 25 percent higher in these people compared to those who got six to nine hours of sleep.

IS POOR SLEEP GETTING IN THE WAY OF A HEALTHY GUT?

Did you know that your gut regenerates its lining while you sleep? Not getting enough sleep may impair the process and may contribute to poor gut health. Getting adequate sleep also gives your gut a chance to get some much-needed R&R. During the day, your gut is typically engaged in near-constant activity. It is enrobed by two rows of neurons: one row is responsible for motility—stretching and squeezing your intestines to push food through the digestive tract—while the other row senses where your food is in the process. Whenever neurons from either row touch, they react automatically to get out of the way. When you're asleep, your busy neurons calm down, which promotes better gut health.

GET YOUR ZZZZZS

At our clinics, we see the link between sleep and food consumption on a daily basis. On days when our patients haven't gotten a good night's sleep, they find it more of a struggle to stick with their eating plan. Just ask Sherri, 37, who lost 18 pounds on the program and has kept it off for four years. She reports, "I was in Week 3 on the Lean for Life program, and I had my cravings pretty much under control, which I was feeling really good about. But then I went out for a girls' night out to celebrate a girlfriend's birthday, and we stayed out way past my normal bedtime. The next morning, I felt like I was starving and wanted to pig out on high-carb foods."

Just like Sherri, we all have nights when we don't sleep well. When you're trying to lose weight, however, it's a good idea to make sleep a priority in your life. Getting seven to eight hours of sleep each night primes your body and brain to melt fat rather than store it. You can help them do their job by following these simple tips for better sleep.

- **Develop a bedtime schedule and stick with it.** Try to hit the hay and wake up at the same time every day of the week—including weekends.

- **Power down.** The artificial light emitted by TVs, computers, smart-phones, tablets, gaming consoles and other screens can disrupt your internal clock. The overstimulation of the brain associated with using these devices can also leave you tossing and turning. Be sure to turn off electronic devices at least one hour before turning in for the night.

- **Take a hot shower.** Raising your body temperature prior to bedtime brings on a sense of relaxation.

- **Exercise, but not before bedtime.** Getting regular physical activity is associated with better sleep, but exercise is energizing—so avoid doing that late-evening Zumba class or doing an interval workout within two hours of bedtime.

- **Have a high PER protein snack.** Protein-rich foods may provide *L-tryptophan*, a snooze-friendly amino acid that is involved in the production of melatonin.

- **Drink something warm.** Sipping on a cup of herbal tea or a hot chocolate protein snack induces sleepiness.

- **Avoid those late-afternoon pick-me-ups.** Drinking a cup of coffee, a glass of iced tea or a shot of an energy drink can help you power through your afternoon but may disrupt your sleep cycle. Limit caffeinated beverages to morning and early afternoon, and stick to decaf or caffeine-free options later in the day and evening.

- **Go with glycine.** Years of research show a connection between the amino acid *glycine* and enhanced sleep quality. According to scientific studies, a supplement made from glycine promotes deeper, sounder and more satisfying sleep. You can find these supplements in drugstores, online and on our website. Getting more deep sleep is critical to feeling refreshed and rejuvenated in the morning.

- **Make friends with magnesium.** Research suggests that magnesium can help you stay asleep throughout the night. Nibble on magnesium-rich foods, such as kelp (seaweed), parsley, shrimp or tofu, or try a magnesium supplement. The recommended dietary allowance is about 300 milligrams per day.

- **Check your DAP.** If you have trouble sleeping, check your DAP to see if you can pinpoint any foods, habits or thoughts that could have led to restless sleep.

DAY 20: MENU DAY

TIME FOR A GUT CHECK

As you've seen throughout this book, your gut plays host to 10 percent of your body's neurons and trillions of bacteria that may have been making it harder for you to lose weight. Today, you'll get a refresher course on the curious roles of gut microflora and discover some simple steps to encourage your gut to continue shrinking those fat cells.

HEALING YOUR GUT

An increasing number of researchers are turning their attention to the gut in hopes of identifying which bugs belong to the enemy forces that make you gain weight and which critters can help you win the battle of the bulge. And they're getting closer to doing so. In one study involving mice, which

The Inside Story from Dr. Allouche

THE BUG BRIGADE

Let's quickly recap what you've learned so far about what's inside your gut and how it affects the size of your waist, hips and thighs.

- More than 100 trillion bugs—some beneficial, some harmful—reside within your gut and may play a role in your eating behaviors and your weight.

- Imbalances in gut microflora can wreak havoc with digestion, cause cravings and may play a role in inflammation, insulin resistance and metabolic syndrome.

- The foods you eat either nourish the beneficial bugs or fuel the bad bacteria. Eating too many foods high in sugar or refined carbohydrates can wipe out many of the beneficial bugs in your digestive tract and lead to problems.

- Your gut plays a role in your immune system, and an overprotective gut may attack certain foods in your digestive tract, leading to an intolerance to those foods.

- Leaky gut, in which the contents of the gut can cross from inside the intestines to the body, can fire up systemic inflammation.

- With 200 million neurons, your gut acts like a second brain in your body, a sort of on-site Mission Control that communicates with the gray matter between your ears to regulate your appetite.

- When your brain, body and gut stop communicating effectively, it wreaks havoc with your satiety.

- Your "second brain" located in your gut produces far more of your body's serotonin than the brain between your ears. Inadequate serotonin levels are associated with depression and a lack of motivation.

have a digestive system similar to our own, scientists discovered that mice lacking a certain type of bacteria didn't gain weight even when they were fed a high-fat diet.

Who knows, in a few years, scientists may develop drugs or vaccines that could destroy the enemy bugs camping out in your gut so the good guys could do a better job of helping you lose weight. Wouldn't that be cool? Until then, rest assured that there are a number of simple strategies you can use to diminish harmful microflora and encourage the growth of friendly gut bacteria.

FEED YOUR FRIENDLY BACTERIA

Prebiotics are fibers in our food that feed, nourish and promote the growth of the friendly bacteria in your gut. These bacteria-fueling fibers include inulin and oligosaccharides. Exciting evidence is showing that consuming prebiotics may help balance blood sugar levels, increase satiety, reduce appetite and ultimately aid in weight loss. You can find prebiotics in many foods, including whole grains, artichokes, asparagus, bananas, onions, endives, leeks, tomatoes and garlic—all foods that get the green light on this program. Look for inulin in fiber supplements and Lean for Life products.

MINIMIZE FOODS THAT FUEL BAD BACTERIA

Reducing your intake of the foods that promote the growth of harmful bacteria can help heal your gut. On this program, you'll be significantly reducing consumption of two of the biggest offenders: sugar and refined carbs. By sticking closely to the menu plans, you can begin to rebalance your gut bacteria to reduce cravings and promote weight loss.

DAY 21: MENU DAY

DISCOVER THE POWER OF pH

Do you remember learning about pH, or "potential of hydrogen," in high school chemistry class? Your pH indicates the level of your body's acidity or alkalinity measured on a scale of 0–14. What does this have to do with getting lean? When the body is too acidic, it drains energy, compromises health and creates an ideal environment for fat to proliferate. Today, we'll show you how increasing alkalinity by eating the alkaline-forming foods recommended on this program reverses these problems and makes it easier to say goodbye to the fat jeans (and genes) and hello to the skinny jeans.

The Inside Story from Dr. Allouche

pH POWER

Decades of scientific research have found that when your body is too acidic, it makes you more vulnerable to weight gain, obesity and type 2 diabetes. It also increases your risk for other problems—such as chronic fatigue, muscle aches and joint pain, and frequent infections—that may indirectly impact your weight. It's no surprise that when you don't have much energy, when you feel achy, or when you feel under the weather from a cold or flu, you are less likely to make the effort to plan and prepare healthy meals, to get your 10,000 steps in or to complete your DAP. When you eat and drink too many acid-forming foods, it creates an acidic buildup that demands your body's attention. Your body has to focus much of its energy on fighting off acidic toxins, which slows down other processes, including your metabolism.

On the other hand, when you include many alkalizing foods in your daily diet, your body can get back to its primary job of optimizing your health and your weight. It's important to understand that you don't need to *eliminate* acid-forming foods to achieve pH balance. As a general rule, you just need to limit some of the most acid-forming foods while making sure to consume alkalizing foods on a regular basis. See "Acid-Forming Foods Limited on Lean for Life" for a list of foods to limit during your program. Rest assured, on this program, you're eating the best foods for tip-top health and rapid weight loss that lasts. On your Menu Days, you're consuming alkalizing foods—such as fruits, vegetables and dark leafy greens—at every meal.

ACID-FORMING FOODS LIMITED ON LEAN FOR LIFE

Proteins: butter, lard, full-fat dairy

Beverages: alcohol, store-bought juices, sweetened sodas, sweetened energy drinks, full-fat cow's milk

Grains: breads, pasta, cereals, refined grains

Legumes: all

Nuts: all

Sweets: sugar, candy, honey, maple syrup, jams, jellies

Other: margarine, mayonnaise

Dr. Stamper Says

THE EASY ANTACID SOLUTION

Dr. Stamper has always been ahead of his time. For as long as I (Cynthia) can remember, he encouraged our family to take measures to avoid an overly acidic system. One simple remedy he prescribed years ago—and still adheres to today—was to add one fourth of a teaspoon of baking soda to a glass of water every day. Many people find this strategy also helps to calm bouts of acidic stomach. I make it a point to add baking soda to the glass of water I drink when I take my supplements each day. It's an easy habit to get into!

HOW ARE YOU MEASURING UP?

As you complete Week 3, this is an ideal time to take stock of your progress. Experts say it takes at least 21 days to form a new habit. Today, on Day 21 of Rapid Weight Loss, you may be close to solidifying some new habits. Is it getting easier to stick with your program, or are you still tempted to go back to your old patterns? Do you feel a bit of a tug of war with your decision-making? Don't worry if you do. Change is challenging. Just remember, your brain is still hard at work laying down and strengthening the new connections that will eventually automate your new habits. In addition, your gut and body are still in the process of being "leanified" so they can help you stay on track, lose weight more easily and then keep it off for good.

In addition to thinking about these internal changes, don't forget to take your measurements today and fill out your "Weekly Progress Report" in Appendix F.

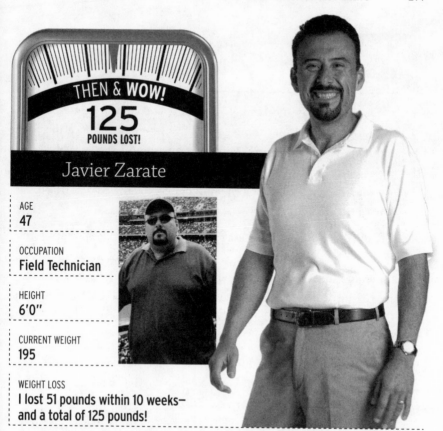

THEN & **WOW!**

125
POUNDS LOST!

Javier Zarate

AGE
47

OCCUPATION
Field Technician

HEIGHT
6'0"

CURRENT WEIGHT
195

WEIGHT LOSS
**I lost 51 pounds within 10 weeks—
and a total of 125 pounds!**

*When I started the Lean for Life program, I weighed 320 pounds. I really
questioned whether it would work for me because I had so much weight to lose.
Making the decision to trust the process and give it 100 percent is the best thing
I ever did. Everything about my life is better since I took control of my weight
and my health.*

DOWNSIZING: I used to wear a 52-inch waist pants and had to shop at
the "Big and Tall" store. These days, I wear a 34-inch waist and can shop
anywhere I want.

TURNING POINT: I knew it was time to do something about my weight
when I was on an airplane and I had to ask for a seat belt extension. That
was so embarrassing and depressing.

LESSONS LEARNED: The Lean for Life program was real education for
me. I not only learned how to eat better, move more and stress less, but

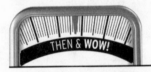

I also learned really practical things like how to overcome a weight plateau and how to make healthier choices at parties where food and drinks are so abundant. I started my program in October and I was nervous that I would struggle through the holidays, but I didn't. I was totally committed. There's something about seeing the number on the scale go down that's very energizing.

TWISTS AND TURNS: I'm a stress eater, and over an especially stressful two-year period, I regained 40 pounds. That was a real wake-up call. It reminded me that maintaining a healthy weight is an ongoing process and that losing the weight is only half the battle. The good news is I know the Lean for Life program works. It's a resource I can always rely on when I need it.

HIT THE SNOOZE BUTTON: Some people look at sleep as wasted time, but I'm a big believer that the eight hours I sleep make the 16 hours I'm awake much more enjoyable. For me, it's a quality of life thing. I just feel so much better when I'm well rested. When I'm fatigued and overtired, it's also way too easy to reach for foods that are loaded with carbs, sugar, fat—and lots of calories I don't want or need.

MR. ENERGY: Before I lost weight, I always felt lazy and tired. Nothing slows me down now. I'm much more productive at work, and I'm much more active with my wife and daughter.

A NEW MAN: People who haven't seen me in a long time sometimes ask my wife if she has a new husband. She definitely does!

RAPID WEIGHT LOSS WEEK 4:

STICKING WITH YOUR PROGRAM WHEN LIFE GETS IN THE WAY

7

Parties, plateaus and other people—these are just a few of the things that can trip up your best intentions, undermine your confidence and stall your progress. Week 4 introduces you to essential solutions—road-tested on *hundreds of thousands* of our patients—for these everyday problems. When you're armed with the right tools, you can handle any situation that arises.

DAY 22: PROTEIN DAY

OVERCOMING PLATEAUS

We have found that for some—but not all—of our patients, the beginning of Week 4 brings a slowing of weight loss. You may think you've hit one of those dreaded plateaus, but not necessarily so. In today's "Inside Story from Dr. Allouche," we'll explore how hormones, cortisol and water retention can *mimic* a plateau, and show you how to determine if what you're experiencing really *is* a plateau. Hint: *not* losing weight while *not* in ketosis is *not* a plateau. If it is the real thing, we'll show you how to shift to our special Plateau Menu for up to three days to reignite weight loss, or you can try our Alternative Menu Plan (AMP) using meal replacements for a few days to amp up results.

YOUR PLATEAU PRIMER

If the number on your scale seems to have gotten stuck, don't be discouraged. Hitting a weight-loss plateau at some point during your program is a common occurrence, even if you're following your program carefully. Your knee-jerk reaction may be to think that you've failed, that this program doesn't work, that you'll never lose any more weight, or that you should just give up and chow down on a double cheeseburger *right now!* Not so fast! We urge you to hit the pause button before you go into panic mode.

We find that when we prepare our patients for the possibility of plateaus and explain what they are, why they happen and what you can do about them, they tend to handle them without getting overly frustrated, taking a hit to their self-confidence or quitting the program. You can benefit from a little plateau preparedness, too.

Some people experience a plateau whenever they return to a weight to which their body is accustomed. Let's look at Emma. She had spent nearly a decade at a weight of 135 before putting on an additional 15 pounds following a stressful divorce. She started her program weighing 150 pounds with a goal weight of 125. Emma dropped 15 pounds quickly, but when she got down to 135, her weight loss stalled. We refer to this type of plateau as "body memory," in which the body achieves a sort of "comfort zone" that it tries to maintain. Scientists have yet to pinpoint exactly why this happens, but our experience over millions of treatment sessions tells us it does indeed happen. The good news is that plateaus are only temporary, usually lasting only one to seven days.

The first thing you need to do when the scale gets stuck is determine whether or not it's a real plateau. Ask yourself the following: Are you in ketosis?

If you're not in ketosis, then you are *not* experiencing a plateau. You're likely consuming too many carbohydrates. Review the last few days of your DAP to see if you can identify the extra carbs. Are you writing down absolutely *everything* you eat and drink on your DAP? Are you reading nutrition labels to make sure you aren't consuming hidden carbs? To get back into ketosis, consider doing one or two Protein Days before resuming your Menu Days.

If you are in ketosis and weight loss has slowed, it still isn't necessarily a plateau. You'll find out why next.

The Inside Story from Dr. Allouche

FAUX PLATEAUS

Did you know that a number of conditions—such as water retention—can mimic a plateau? We call these *faux plateaus*. That's because you may still be losing fat, but because you're retaining water, the scale doesn't reflect your progress. And since water weighs more than fat, it's even possible to be losing fat while retaining water and have the scale reflect a weight *gain*. Rest assured, there are simple strategies you can use to reverse water retention and to see your scale start cooperating again. Before we share them with you, let's take a look at some of the causes of water retention.

- **Hormonal fluctuations:** Many women experience water retention as a symptom of pre-menstrual syndrome (PMS). When women are going through peri-menopause or menopause, water retention may become chronic.

- **Elevated stress hormone levels:** Stress hormones, such as cortisol, promote water retention—the more stress you've got, the more water you hold on to. Stress can come from everyday aggravation, financial problems, relationship woes and more.

- **Consuming too much sodium:** Did you know that every salt molecule in your body attracts two water molecules? This explains why too much sodium in the diet increases fluid retention and could be causing your faux plateau. Check your DAP to see if you've been adding too much salt to your food or eating too many salty snacks or processed foods, which tend to have loads of sodium.

- **Consuming too many carbs:** In terms of water retention, molecules of glucose (carbohydrate) act like salt molecules. Each and every glucose molecule inside your body attracts two molecules of water. Ingesting too many carbs increases the amount of water and may cause your scale to get stuck. Review your DAP to determine if you're consuming too many carbs.

FAUX PLATEAU BUSTERS

In our clinics, we have helped thousands and thousands of patients recognize faux plateaus and eliminate them so they can get back on track with Rapid Weight Loss. Here are some simple strategies to reduce water retention that we share with our patients. They may help you, too.

- **Step away from the salt shaker.** If you typically season your food with salt, don't! Grab the pepper shaker instead. Eliminate salty snacks and reduce your intake of processed foods. Be aware that some beverages may contain sodium, too. Make it a habit to check all nutrition labels for sodium content before consuming anything.

- **Add potassium to your plate.** Potassium reduces fluid retention, so be sure to eat potassium-rich foods, including bananas, spinach, non-fat yogurt, salmon and white mushrooms on your Menu Days.

- **Drink more water.** It may seem counter-intuitive, but guzzling more H_2O can be one of the best ways to flush out excess water.

- **Break a sweat.** Regular exercise can drain stored water and excess salt through perspiration.

- **De-stress.** Practicing the deep breathing, meditation and sleep recommendations presented in this book can reduce cortisol levels, which will help with fluid balance.

- **Try natural diuretics.** Regular black tea is a safe, natural diuretic that will work for you if you are not a regular user of caffeine. You may also want to try boiling a cup of water with a quarter of a lemon (including the rind) and drinking the hot lemon water to obtain a mild diuretic effect. *Warning: Do not take any pharmaceutical diuretics unless prescribed by your physician.*

If the simple strategies described here don't work, try the "Plateau Menu" for *no more than three days* or until you "break" the plateau by losing 1 ½ pounds or more, whichever comes first. If you prefer, you can try our AMP (see "AMP Menu Plan" on page 184) using meal replacements for a few days to reignite weight loss. In Appendix A, you will find a "DAP for AMP" sheet along with a few FAQs about this plateau-busting plan.

PLATEAU MENU

BREAKFAST

1 Egg or egg substitute (boiled, poached or cooked with cooking spray in a nonstick pan)

½ Grapefruit

1 Calorie-free beverage

MID-MORNING SNACK

1 Protein OR 1 Lean for Life Protein Snack

LUNCH

3½ Ounces white fish

½ Cup cooked spinach

1 Cup lettuce

½ Grapefruit

1 Calorie-free beverage

MID-AFTERNOON SNACK

1 Protein OR 1 Lean for Life Protein Snack

DINNER

3½ Ounces white fish

½ Cup cooked spinach

1 Cup lettuce

½ Grapefruit

1 Calorie-free beverage

EVENING SNACK

1 Protein OR 1 Lean for Life Protein Snack

continued

PLATEAU MENU

BEDTIME

1 Cup hot lemon water (¼ lemon boiled in water for 3 minutes)

AMP MENU PLAN

BREAKFAST

2 Liquid proteins

LUNCH

2 Liquid proteins

MID-AFTERNOON SNACK

1 High PER protein bar

DINNER

1 Protein

1 Vegetable

1 Fruit

EVENING SNACK

1 Liquid protein

DAY 23: MENU DAY

THE ABC'S—PLUS THE D'S, E'S AND MORE—OF VITAMINS AND SUPPLEMENTS

Is there such a thing as weight loss from a pill? While there are no magic pills that can instantly and safely melt fat, certain vitamins and supplements can enhance your weight-loss progress in a variety of ways. If you've been following this program carefully, you're already taking the recommended vitamins and supplements. Today, we're going to fill you in on the reasons why it's so important to take them throughout the 28 days of the Rapid Weight Loss phase of the program and beyond.

When you reduce the number of calories you consume, you also reduce the amount of nutrients you get from food. Plus, on this program, you may lose water, which means you're also losing water-soluble vitamins and minerals. For these reasons, it is critical that you replace what you've lost to ensure that you're getting an adequate amount of nutrients. We've developed our own multivitamins that have been specially formulated to provide you with what you need while on this program. If you prefer to choose another brand of vitamins, be sure to look for one that provides comparable dosages.

Let's take a look at some of the most important vitamins and supplements that may be beneficial to you while you're getting leaner.

BEEF UP YOUR B VITAMINS

If you want to leap out of bed raring to go in the morning, power through cold season without the sniffles, keep stress under control, remember where you left your car keys and optimize metabolism, you've gotta get your Bs. The B vitamins—thiamine (B_1), riboflavin (B_2), niacin (B_3), pantothenic acid (B_5), pyroxidine (B_6), cyanocobalamine (B_{12}), folic acid and biotin—are critical nutrients for a vast array of bodily functions, but the one you're probably most interested in is the ability to metabolize fats, carbohydrates and protein for energy. B_{12} is the most important of the B vitamins involved in the fat-burning process.

B vitamins help the weight-loss process in another way, too—by increasing the absorption and use of protein by muscle cells. This is especially important when following a high-protein diet that results in rapid weight loss. When people lose weight on this program, they lose mostly fat, but there also may be some muscle loss. The B vitamins, especially B_6, help minimize muscle loss. When you're eating a high-protein diet, it increases your need for B_6. In a study from a team of Japanese researchers published in the *Journal of Nutritional Science and Vitaminology,* rats fed a 70 percent protein diet needed twice the amount of B_6 as rats getting only 20 percent of their food from protein. Without the extra B_6, the rats didn't grow optimally, and their lean tissues were deficient in B_6.

Lean for Life–approved foods that are high in B vitamins are as follows:
- Dark green leafy vegetables
- Chicken, beef, turkey, fish, shellfish, eggs
- Whole grains
- Bananas

SEE THE SUPER BENEFITS OF VITAMIN C

Vitamin C is indispensable for human life. In addition to its well-known benefits, including boosting immunity, fighting fatigue and synthesizing red blood cells, vitamin C may play a role in inflammation and weight gain. Some research suggests that a lack of vitamin C is pro-inflammatory, which, as you've learned in this book, is associated with increased fat storage. Most animals are capable of making their own vitamin C internally, but humans lack this ability and must get this antioxidant through food and other sources.

When you restrict your intake of food as you're doing on this program, you may not be getting enough vitamin C from your diet, so it's a good idea to supplement your intake.

Lean for Life–approved foods that are high in vitamin C are as follows:
- Dark green leafy vegetables
- Red bell peppers
- Papayas
- Strawberries
- Kiwi
- Cantaloupe
- Citrus fruits

CAN VITAMIN D AID IN WEIGHT LOSS?

The "sunshine vitamin" does a lot more than improve bone health, boost moods and shore up immunity. A growing body of evidence suggests that low levels of this vitamin could be what makes that number on the scale keep going higher and higher. For a 2012 study in the *Journal of Women's Health,* researchers followed more than 4,600 women aged 65 and over for four and a half years. They found that those with insufficient levels of vitamin D gained more weight than those with adequate levels of the vitamin. Other research suggests that increasing vitamin D levels when starting a weight-loss program may result in better results. You can also increase vitamin D levels by getting 10 to 20 minutes of sunshine a day.

Lean for Life–approved foods that are high in vitamin D are as follows:
- Fish
- Fortified cereals
- Fortified soy products
- Fortified fat-free dairy
- Eggs
- Mushrooms

PUMP UP POTASSIUM

Your body needs the mineral potassium to build muscle, maintain proper electrolyte balance, control your heart's electrical activity, and break down and use carbohydrates for energy. This powerful substance can also improve blood pressure and reduce fatigue, stress and headaches. A significant reduction in calorie intake may result in potassium deficiency, and weight loss can reduce the enzyme activity that controls the flow of potassium and sodium by 20 percent, so it is especially important to take supplemental potassium while on this program.

Symptoms of low potassium levels include muscle weakness, muscle cramps, fatigue or lack of energy. Note that these same symptoms may also be caused by dehydration due to inadequate fluid intake. Severe potassium deficiency can cause serious consequences, such as irregularities in heart rhythm. In addition to taking a high-quality multivitamin and mineral supplement during this program, our clinic patients take a prescription-strength oral potassium chloride supplement (750 mg/10 mEq) to maintain healthy potassium levels. Potassium is also available over the counter in lower doses in the form of potassium gluconate. Table salt and salt substitutes also contain potassium. (*Important: If you are being treated for chronic disease, high blood pressure or are taking potassium-sparing diuretics, you should not take extra potassium supplements without first consulting your primary health-care provider.*)

Lean for Life–approved foods that are high in potassium are as follows:
- Meats, poultry and fish
- Soy products
- Vegetables (broccoli, spinach, tomatoes, zucchini)
- Fruits (especially citrus, bananas, kiwi and cantaloupe)
- Nonfat dairy

MUST-KNOW INFO ON MAGNESIUM

Did you know that up to 80 percent of Americans may not be getting the recommended daily allowance of magnesium? This is bad news, considering that every organ in your body and every bodily process needs an adequate intake of this mineral for optimal functioning. When you're losing weight, magnesium takes on even more importance. That's because magnesium is heavily involved in helping your body digest, absorb, and use proteins, carbohydrates, and fats. You can also thank it for helping insulin usher glucose into your cells for energy. Known as the anti-stress mineral, magnesium also plays a role in keeping the fat-promoting hormone cortisol under control and improves sleep.

Other potential health benefits of magnesium include reduced risk for type 2 diabetes, protection against osteoporosis, healthier blood pressure levels and reduced risk for heart disease. In fact, new evidence is revealing that magnesium is absolutely critical for heart health. In a 2013 study appearing in the *American Journal of Clinical Nutrition,* researchers from the Netherlands checked the magnesium levels of 7,664 healthy people and then tracked them for an average of at least 10 years. The study's findings were startling: people with the lowest levels of magnesium were 70 percent more likely to die from heart disease than people with higher levels. The encouraging news from this study is that researchers suggest that simply increasing your intake of the mighty mineral could reduce the risk of heart disease. If you don't like taking supplements, you can now find magnesium in the form of lotions and serums.

Lean for Life–approved foods that are high in magnesium are as follows:
- Green leafy vegetables
- Whole grains
- Nonfat dairy
- Soy products
- Bananas
- Apricots

WHAT'S SELENIUM GOT TO DO WITH SLIMMING?

A powerful antioxidant, selenium supports healthy thyroid function, which is key for metabolism. When the thyroid gland isn't functioning properly, a condition called *hypothyroidism,* it can lead to weight gain.

Lean for Life–approved foods that are high in selenium are as follows:
- Beef, poultry, eggs, fish
- Whole grains

HOW IRON HELPS YOU MOVE MORE

Iron's primary job is to help your red blood cells shuttle oxygen throughout your body. Iron deficiency, known as *anemia*, means that cells are not getting the oxygen they need. This will leave you feeling tired and listless. When you feel fatigued, it makes it more difficult for you to engage in the physical activity that fuels weight loss.

Lean for Life–approved foods that are high in iron are as follows:
- Beef
- Turkey
- Spinach

SHRINKING FAT CELLS WITH OMEGA-3 FATTY ACIDS?

Omega-3 fatty acids have long been touted for their positive effects on heart health, brain function and mood stabilization, as well as for their anti-inflammatory properties. Low levels of these essential fatty acids have been linked to a greater risk for obesity, which has sparked a flurry of research into the possibility of increasing omega-3 intake as a potential weight-loss aid.

Research has been mixed, but some studies have shown a positive effect. For example, Australian researchers reported in a 2013 issue of *Food & Function* that women taking omega-3 fish oil supplements while dieting lost more weight than dieters who took a placebo. Another study from the same team of researchers appearing in the *British Journal of Nutrition* in 2012 showed different results. In this trial, which compared weight loss among people taking omega-3 supplements or a placebo, the research team found that although omega-3 supplementation while dieting did not produce a significant difference in the amount of weight lost, it did produce a significant increase in the reduction of body fat compared to those taking a placebo. Losing more body fat equals getting leaner, so to us that sounds like a positive result.

Lean for Life–approved foods that are high in omega-3 fatty acids are as follows:
- Halibut, salmon, scallops, shrimp, tuna
- Eggs (DHA-enriched)

FUN FACTS ABOUT FIBER

Decades of research confirm that consuming a diet high in fiber helps control appetite, which can help speed your way to a leaner physique. Scientists are now beginning to understand how it works—consuming fiber decreases levels of the appetite hormone ghrelin to keep you feeling full longer. In addition, some fibers, such as inulin, are prebiotics that promote healthy gut bacteria. Eating high-fiber foods is one way to tap into the benefits of fiber, but taking a fiber supplement can be helpful, too. In fact, a 2008 study in the *British Journal of Nutrition* found that people taking a fiber supplement lost more weight than those who didn't.

Lean for Life–approved foods that are high in fiber are as follows:
- Vegetables
- Fruits
- Whole grains and fortified cereals

GIMME SOME GAMMA-LINOLENIC ACID

Gamma-linolenic acid (GLA) is an omega-6 fatty acid that may be a key component in successful weight management. Clinical evidence suggests that GLA may suppress weight regain following major weight loss. GLA is currently available in supplement form. Lean for Life's Stay-Weight Dietary Supplement contains the most concentrated source of GLA commercially available.

CAPSINOIDS: A NATURAL METABOLISM BOOSTER

Say hello to a natural supplement called CH-19, derived from a rare sweet pepper variety that has been shown in numerous clinical studies to increase metabolism and promote fat-burning *without* increasing heart rate or blood pressure. The CH-19 sweet pepper is rich in a substance called capsinoids, which are similar to capsaicin, the pungent element that gives hot chili peppers their heat. Lean for Life's Capsio-Lin provides this supplement, which clinical studies indicate may naturally increase your metabolism.

The Inside Story from Dr. Allouche

ARE YOU GETTING THE MOST FROM YOUR VITAMINS AND SUPPLEMENTS?

Did you know that you could be taking vitamins faithfully but not getting the benefits you expect? Your age, gender, dietary habits and overall health play a role in your ability to absorb the nutrients in supplements. In addition, the way some supplements are manufactured can enhance or reduce what's known as their "bio-availability," or the ability to be absorbed by the body. Unfortunately, in some cases, when you swallow a vitamin, your stomach acids attack it and reduce its bio-availability. When this happens, those expensive vitamins exit your body every time you urinate. Talk about throwing your money down the toilet... *literally!*

When it comes to vitamins and supplements, make sure you're getting the most bang for your buck by choosing products that have the highest levels of bio-availability. Look for products that come in gel caps or that have an enteric coating, as they tend to stand up better to the stomach's harsh acids. Vitamin injections, which are available in many physicians' offices and pharmacies, are another delivery option that is highly bio-available.

DAY 24: MENU DAY

COOK UP A HEALTHIER LIFE

As you near the end of your 28-day Rapid Weight Loss phase of the program, you may start worrying about what comes next and how you'll manage to keep the weight off. Our years of clinical experience have taught us that certain ingredients are essential for a healthier life. On this day, we'll share our "recipe" for lasting success.

TO YOUR "HEALTH"

All you need is a healthy dose of "HEALTH" to keep living life the lean way. HEALTH stands for:

Higher purpose

Eating better

Activity on a regular basis

Laughter and play

Time alone

Human contact

HIGHER PURPOSE

You may wonder what having a higher purpose has to do with becoming Lean for Life. We have found that among our patients, those who have a sense of purpose and passion in life tend to maintain their weight loss. Those who feel a connection to something greater than themselves not only feel more fulfilled but they also feel more of a sense of accountability for their actions. When you feel like your life matters, then you're likely to feel more of an obligation to treat yourself and your body with respect. Spiritual beliefs, commitment to a cause or ideals, and participation in activities that inspire you can activate the pleasure center of your brain in much healthier ways than the overindulgence of food. What matters to you? What stirs your passions? Find your passions and follow them.

EATING BETTER

Although you are currently in the Rapid Weight Loss phase of this program, your ultimate goal is to develop healthy eating habits that will last a lifetime so you can become Lean for Life. As you are learning, the emphasis is on lean protein, vegetables and fruits, whole grains, and healthy dairy options. After you achieve your weight loss, you'll see the benefits of continuing to focus on the healthy eating habits that got you to your goal.

ACTIVITY ON A REGULAR BASIS

Sticking to the physical activity habit you've been developing since Day 1 of this program—whether it's walking at a moderate pace, doing 90-second fat-burning intervals, adding more NEAT into your life or all of the above—provides a laundry list of benefits that promote a healthy weight and a healthy outlook on life.

LAUGHTER AND PLAY

When we laugh, our bodies work better, our relationships work better and our careers work better. Not only does a good laugh feel good, it *does* good. Laughter is one of the ultimate BioModifiers—it nurtures the soul, relieves stress, boosts moods and releases "Leandorphins" that make you feel great. Setting aside a little playtime for fun can do wonders to help you cope with life's challenges. Learning to laugh at yourself and not take yourself so seriously can help you flip the switch on negativity and strengthen a positive attitude that will serve you well.

TIME ALONE

In our chaotic, ever-connected culture, finding some alone time isn't easy, and to be honest, it isn't really encouraged. What a shame! Solitude gives your brain and body a chance to unwind, relax and reflect. There is an emotional clarity and inner calm that can occur only when we're alone, reflecting and thinking without interruption.

When you hop off life's treadmill for some alone time every now and then, it gives you a chance to recharge the spirit and renew your sense of wonder and joy in life. When was the last time you spent a quiet afternoon alone, with no internet, no TV and no rules? Schedule time alone the same way you would schedule a business appointment or lunch meeting. Put it on your calendar and keep your appointment with yourself.

HUMAN CONTACT

Humans are social animals, and we need to connect with other people on a meaningful level for the sake of our well-being. Companionship, it appears, can be good medicine, too. According to a review of more than 148 studies on the subject, researchers concluded that a robust social network may be as important to your long-term health as not smoking. Having close friendships also fends off depression and increases support of healthy habits. Make it a habit to seek out good friends on a regular basis.

Week 4 is a good time to start shifting your focus to these ingredients for a healthier life. If any of these areas in your life could use a little more attention, start taking the time to treat yourself well. "HEALTH" is an investment in yourself. And like any good investment, it will pay off over the long term.

The Inside Story from Dr. Allouche

COOK UP HEALTHIER EATING HABITS

As you read previously, eating better is one of the ingredients of cooking up a healthier life after you reach the end of this program. Throughout this book, you've been learning ways to eat better so you can become Lean for Life. Here, you're going to discover several scientifically based tips to help you continue to make the best choices going forward.

CHEW! CHEW!

Did you know that compared to lean people, obese individuals tend to chew their food fewer times before swallowing it? It's easy to understand the connection between obesity and gulping. As you saw in chapter 1, where you followed a slice of pizza as it takes an amazing journey through your digestive system, when you gulp down your food, your brain and gut don't have enough time to produce enough of the satiety hormones that indicate fullness. That's why even if you've just eaten a double-decker burger and fries, you may still feel ravenous and continue to eat more. Don't think the burger chains don't know this. They do. They clearly understand that finely ground beef and airy white buns as opposed to lean steak and whole grains are much easier to gobble up quickly and that doing so will encourage you to eat a second or even a third burger despite their sky-high calorie and fat content.

Chewing your food more times is the answer. One study showed that when people chewed their food 40 times, they ate nearly 12 percent less than when they chewed only 15 times. In addition, chewing longer sparked an almost immediate reduction in hunger hormones, so they felt fuller faster.

What's your chew quotient? How many times do you chew your food before swallowing? At your next meal, eat the way you normally do and count the number of times you chew before swallowing. Also take note of your level of satiety after this meal. The following time you eat make it a point to chew your food 40 times before swallowing and notice the difference in how quickly you feel full.

FOLLOW THE 20-MINUTE RULE

When it's time to eat, take at least 20 minutes to complete your meal. Why? As you've already seen, when you eat protein, special peptides in the protein saturate nearby mu-opioid receptors in the portal vein, which send satiety signals to the brain to keep you feeling full for more than four hours. It takes 20 minutes for this important digestive process to take place. To gain the maximum benefit from these powerful peptides, allow at least 20 minutes for eating.

EAT LEAN PROTEIN TO GET LEANER

If you want to remain Lean for Life, continue to choose lean proteins that are low in saturated fats and opt for healthy high PER protein snacks that are low in calories, sugar and carbs.

CONTINUE TO USE THE GI AS YOUR GUIDE

As a general rule, making the majority of your meals with foods that are low GI (below 55) will increase satiety, reduce cravings and keep you lean.

COOK YOUR CARBS AL DENTE

Beware! Those whole grains such as whole-wheat pasta and brown rice that rank low to moderate on the glycemic index may not actually be that low—*depending on how you cook them!* If you overcook them until they're mushy, their glycemic index jumps from about 35 for whole-wheat pasta and 50 for brown rice all the way up to about 90, which is almost as high as table sugar!

To keep their GI low, cook whole-grain carbs *al dente*. In Italian, "al dente" literally means "to the tooth," which translates to "firm but not hard when you bite into it." When cooking at home or dining out, always go al dente. It will help keep insulin and blood sugar levels in check, which will help get your waistline in check.

EAT BREAKFAST

Did you eat breakfast this morning? It's a habit shared by 78 percent of the successful dieters being tracked by the National Weight Control Registry (NWCR). The NWCR keeps tabs on the habits of dieters who have lost 30 pounds or more and kept it off for at least one year. Other studies show that people who begin their day with a healthy breakfast are better able to control their calorie intake throughout the rest of the day.

In addition to providing energy and nutrition, breakfast also helps moderate appetite, which makes it easier to avoid mid-day munchies and binges. Eating a healthy breakfast also jump-starts your metabolism to increase fat burning. Breakfast also benefits your brain as well as your body; studies reveal that those who eat breakfast do better on cognitive tests than those who skip breakfast.

MAKE FRIENDS WITH YOUR AMINO AMIGOS

As previously discussed, amino acids are the building blocks of protein in the human body. These "amino amigos" are responsible for much of the repair and rebuilding that takes place within your organs, cells and muscles. Your body can produce some, but not all, of the more than 20 types of amino acids on its own. There are eight amino acids, called the essential amino acids, that must be supplied by food. Your body cannot store excess amino acids the way it stores excess carbohydrates and fats for later use, which means that you need a daily supply of essential amino acids for optimal functioning.

Which foods provide all eight of the essential amino acids? Animal proteins, such as meat, eggs and dairy, are considered *complete* proteins, whereas the proteins derived from most vegetables, grains and other sources lack certain amino acids. When you're taking in fewer calories and aren't eating enough complete proteins, your body is going to look for those essential amino acids somewhere. Usually, it robs tissues from your muscles in order to get the amino acids it needs, leaving you with withered muscles and slower metabolism.

When choosing protein snacks, look for ones that contain all the essential amino acids. This will help you maintain muscle mass, which enhances metabolism and helps keep you Lean for Life.

BECOME A LEAN SHOPPER

A trip to the grocery store can open up a world of temptation. Grocers have spent years and hundreds of millions of dollars mastering the art of marketing to entice you to buy foods and beverages that will make you pack on the pounds.

Arm yourself with the following strategies:

- Use the "Lean for Life Shopping List" (see page 59).
- Shop less often.
- Shop for fresh and frozen fruits and veggies.
- Beware of misleading buzzwords like "Gluten-free" or "No sugar added."
- Learn to read nutrition labels.

DAY 25: MENU DAY

ARE YOUR FRIENDS MAKING YOU GAIN WEIGHT?

Did you know that if you have a sibling or a spouse who is obese, your risk of becoming obese increases by about 40 percent, and if you have a friend who is obese, your risk skyrockets by 57 percent? That's according to data culled from a decades-long health study called the Framingham Heart Study. Yikes! That's *not* what friends are for! Girls' night out, Monday Night Football with the guys, happy hour with coworkers—these are potential diet killers. Fortunately, we can help you put on some "training wheels" by showing you how to safely navigate social situations using something called "episodic future thinking." Research shows that people who use this simple technique are less inclined to overeat in tempting situations.

EPISODIC FUTURE THINKING—WHAT YOU SEE IS WHAT YOU GET

Episodic future thinking may sound like science fiction, but it's actually a very basic concept that's akin to mental time travel or mental rehearsal in which you "pre-experience" a future event. The scientific findings on it indicate that identifying long-term goals and imagining yourself achieving those goals increases their saliency or importance. And in moments of temptation, imagining reaching those goals may improve impulse control.

Here's how this concept might play out. Let's say you're at lunch with two coworkers, and they both order a bacon cheeseburger with fries. You're tempted to say, "Make it three!" But then you pause and imagine yourself zipping up your skinny jeans as you get ready for a night on the town. You really feel the denim comfortably hugging—not squeezing—your hips, and you envision yourself gazing into a mirror and seeing your leaner physique in those jeans. And you like what you see! Then it's back to reality in the restaurant with your coworkers, and you order a spinach salad with grilled chicken and vinaigrette on the side. Temptation thwarted!

This same concept goes for when you're tempted to bail out on your physical activity. When you're getting ready for your early-morning walk, and your walking buddy sends a text saying she's got the sniffles and can't make it, it can be too easy to throw in the towel and go back to bed. Instead, if you imagine how energized you will feel after you finish your walk, you'll be inspired to get out there and hit the road rather than heading back to your bedroom to hit the hay.

Strengthening your episodic future thinking skills will help keep you on track not only to reach your goal weight but also to maintain your weight loss. Start practicing this powerful technique today. By pre-experiencing these benefits of becoming Lean for Life, you're more likely to achieve them.

- Imagine yourself looking leaner and wearing a favorite pair of jeans, dress, bikini, bathing trunks or business suit.

- Envision yourself reaching the finish line of a 5K charity walk or reaching the top of a local hiking trail.

- Think about walking into a room full of strangers and feeling totally confident about yourself and the way you look.

- Imagine waking up bursting with energy.

The Inside Story from Dr. Allouche

HOW FRIENDS MAKE YOU GAIN WEIGHT

Intrigued by the findings of the Framingham Heart Study data, researchers at Arizona State University wanted to delve more deeply into the ways your social network influences your weight. To do so, they recruited 112 women, half of whom were overweight or obese, and then contacted 812 of their friends, family and coworkers. They tested three different possible ways that their relationships with overweight friends could impact their own weight.

- **Bulldozing:** Let's say your overweight friends think it's normal to be overweight or obese. In conversations with them, they bully you into adopting their beliefs about weight, eating and exercise. For instance, they might say, "Everyone gains weight during menopause. There's nothing you can do about it. Here, have a cupcake; it will make you feel better about it." Eventually you may come to share those beliefs and alter your behavior to achieve the same weight as your friends.

- **Internalizing:** In this scenario, even if you don't have direct conversations with your overweight friends about weight, you may internalize their beliefs and subsequently change your behaviors until your body size matches theirs.

- **Mirroring:** You may not share your overweight friends' ideas about normal body size, but you mirror their eating and exercise behaviors and wind up looking like them anyway. For example, if you vow not to eat any dessert after dinner, but then you go out with friends and every single one of them orders a piece of cheesecake for dessert, you end up ordering one, too. That's mirroring. Nobody bulldozed you into ordering cheesecake, and you know that you don't want to be overweight like your friends, but you go with the flow anyway.

Which one of these three ways do you think turned out to be the most likely to have an influence on a person's weight? Mirroring. In fact, mirroring the behaviors of overweight or obese friends was the *only* one of the three ways that showed an impact on body size.

This reinforces what you have been learning throughout this book—it is your behaviors and habits that largely determine your weight. By using the strategies presented in this book, you can automate healthy habits of eating better, moving more and stressing less so you are less inclined to mirror the behaviors of those around you.

DAY 26: MENU DAY

BE AN ACTOR

In some social situations, it may be beneficial to pretend that you are *not* following a diet program. Why? Because we've learned that when our patients tell friends about their new diet, many of these so-called "friends" try to sabotage their efforts. We've also learned that our patients have their own "Inner Committee" of saboteurs inside their heads that can also get in the way of success. Today, we'll show you the secrets to getting lean without appearing to be on a program, we'll show you how to take charge of your inner committee, and in today's "Inside Story from Dr. Allouche," we'll introduce you to the power of mental rehearsal, a mental training technique that allows you to fool your own brain so you can successfully navigate any situation.

FRIENDS AND SABOTEURS

It's a sad fact, but sometimes, friends don't want you to succeed in becoming Lean for Life. Why not? Often, it's because they feel bad about their own weight, and seeing you get leaner just makes them feel worse about it. And that's when the sabotage begins. Imagine this scenario: you and your overweight friend pass by a doughnut shop and she says, "Let's stop and get a doughnut." You politely decline, explaining that you've lost 18 pounds on the Lean for Life program and are feeling fantastic—but instead of expressing support for your progress, she rolls her eyes and says, "Oh, c'mon, one little doughnut won't hurt." Or you're at a dinner party and even though you told your hosts that you've been losing weight on your program and would appreciate eating light, they overload your plate with way too much food. What do you do?

It's time to be an actor and start fooling your friends so they stop messing with your success. Try these tactics to avoid the sabotage scenario.

- **When they won't take "no" for an answer.** What if your host insists that you have a piece of cake? Take the plate and thank her profusely. Then, when she turns away, give it to your spouse, give half to another friend or discreetly dump it in the trash. What if your dinner host puts too much food on your plate? Eat the proper amount then push the food around your plate so it looks like you ate almost everything.

- **Don't be afraid to leave something on your plate.** If your host or hostess wonders if you didn't like the meal, reassure him or her that it was absolutely delicious but say that you ate a late lunch and weren't very hungry.

- **Stick with one drink.** If it's a festive occasion and you want to participate in the toast, accept one glass of champagne and nurse it throughout the night. You can even add water to your champagne glass. If your host tries to pour wine for you with dinner, say you want to stick with champagne.

- **Prepare your excuses beforehand.** Have a plan for any possible sabotage situations and remember that telling a little white lie now and then is worth it if it helps you become Lean for Life.

WHO'S IN CHARGE OF YOUR INNER COMMITTEE?

Leslie was cruising along with her weight loss and then hit a minor plateau in Week 4 and started doubting her ability to reach her goal. She started wondering if she should just give up on her program entirely.

Marcus dropped weight quickly at first—9 pounds in the first week—but then the weight started coming off a bit more slowly. Even though he still dropped a few pounds in Week 4, he started beating himself up because he wasn't losing it fast enough. He felt like a failure and wondered if he even deserved to become Lean for Life.

Andrea was thrilled that she had lost 13 pounds so far and was more than halfway to her goal weight. But on some days, in spite of her success, she would question whether her goal was really worth the effort and whether she had what it takes to maintain her weight loss.

Like Leslie, Marcus and Andrea, you may experience an array of contradictory emotions on your journey to becoming Lean for Life. We like to say that becoming Lean for Life is like a marathon, not a sprint. And like marathon runners, there are days during training when you'll feel like you can't go on or you'll wonder if it's worth all the effort. But we can tell you that when marathon runners reach that finish line, they know that every minute of sweat equity they put into reaching their goal was worth it. You will, too.

As you continue to work toward your goal, be prepared to listen to a number of conflicting voices inside your head, all competing to be heard. One of your inner voices is loving and supportive. Another is harsh and critical.

There's even a curious, playful one. Each of those voices has a point of view and an agenda. We call these voices your "Inner Committee," and you absolutely must assume the role of chairperson of that committee.

Perhaps you recognize some or all of these common voices, and you may have some of your own to add to the list. Do any of these sound familiar?

- **Your frightened voice:** *I'm afraid I'm not going to do this right.*
- **Your angry voice:** *I'm never allowed to do or say what I want!*
- **Your critical voice:** *Don't even bother—you don't deserve it.*
- **Your joyful voice:** *Hey, let's do this! This is wonderful!*
- **Your curious voice:** *I'll figure out a way to do this!*
- **Your loving voice:** *I'm with you, no matter what!*
- **Your confident voice:** *I can do it!*

Considering all these different voices vying for control, it's no wonder you may feel confident one day and critical the next day, or even joyful in the afternoon and then frightened just a few hours later. Understanding that these apparent contradictions are a normal part of the process can help you develop a balanced perspective on your inner conflicts. It can also remind you that whatever voice is speaking at any particular moment isn't the only voice you have.

Think of your Inner Committee as a Board of Directors in which all members offer their own individual opinions and insights. You wouldn't let any one Board member tell you what to do, would you? Of course not. You would let all the members weigh in and then, based on all the information you've received, you would do what you've decided is in your best interest.

Try this exercise to gain control of your Inner Committee. "Sit in" on a meeting of your Inner Committee. Write down what your different voices are saying, as well as your responses to them. Make note of the negative comments you're hearing or feeling, but focus primarily on what your loving, joyful, curious and confident voices say to counter negative messages. Cultivate strong, positive voices so they can overpower the negative ones.

The Inside Story from Dr. Allouche

THE POWER OF MENTAL REHEARSAL

Years ago, motivational speaker Zig Ziglar wrote about a prisoner of war (POW) during the war in Vietnam who survived his horrid conditions by playing a mental round of golf every day. The POW, who had been a recreational golfer prior to his imprisonment, created a golf course in his mind and would visualize every stroke and every time the ball rolled into the hole. According to the story, when the POW was finally released and returned home to the United States, he headed to the nearest golf course, where he proceeded to knock 20 strokes off his average. This reveals the power of the human mind using a mental training technique known as mental rehearsal.

Mental rehearsal activates neural pathways associated with the skill or activity being imagined. This appears to strengthen these pathways in much the same way that physical practice does. For years, sports psychologists have advocated the use of mental rehearsal to improve athletic skills. You can take advantage of this simple mental training technique to help you master your behavior in a variety of situations.

It's easy. Let's say you're invited to a wedding, and you're fretting that your willpower won't stand up to the enticing buffet and five-tier wedding cake. Take a few moments and mentally practice what you'll do. Imagine yourself walking into the reception and a server approaching you with a plate full of cheese-filled pastry-puff hors d'oeuvres. Experience the mouth-watering smell of the melted cheese and the flaky pastry wafting your way. Then imagine yourself saying, "No, thank you" and continuing your conversation with your date.

See yourself strolling over to the bar to order a glass of sparkling water with a twist of lime. Mentally practice your approach to the buffet. See yourself bypassing the roasted potatoes, bread rolls, and Ranch dressing-doused salad and instead taking a small portion of delicious lean protein and heading back to your seat. Continue your mental rehearsal, imagining the server planting a slice of cake in front of you and see yourself immediately handing it back with a quick, "No, thanks." Keep practicing, and when the big day comes, you'll be hardwired to do the right thing.

Here are some keys to getting the most out of mental rehearsal:

- **Eliminate distractions:** Find a quiet place where you can practice mental rehearsal.

- **Use all of your senses:** Smell the fresh-baked bread rolls, hear the crunch when your date bites into a cracker topped with cheese and feel the cold glass of refreshing sparkling water in your hand.

- **Rehearse often:** The more you practice, the more likely you are to follow through the way you visualized your behavior.

DAY 27: MENU DAY

THE POWER OF PRACTICE

Have you ever considered all the "practice" you had to do in order to learn the habits that caused you to become overweight? Probably not. You're more likely to feel like you just woke up one day and—boom!—none of your clothes fit anymore. But the reality is that you repeatedly trained your brain, body and gut to adopt the kind of habits that make you gain weight.

OLD UNHEALTHY HABITS

- Overindulge—repeat nightly.
- Make poor food choices—repeat 3–5 times per day.
- Sit on the couch—at least 4 hours per day.
- Feel bad, eat pizza, feel better—after every disagreement with your spouse, coworkers or friends.
- Want ice cream, eat ice cream—whenever the mood strikes.

By the same token, the past 26 days have served as practice for creating habits that will make you Lean for Life. By now, changes in your neuronal pathways are already taking place. Today we're going to focus on one of the habits that may have gotten you into trouble in the past and hone in on the continued practice that will strengthen your newly laid connections to help you break that habit and replace it with new ones.

WHAT'S THE PROBLEM WITH "I WANT IT, AND I WANT IT NOW"?

It's midnight, and you wake up with a monster craving for chunky fudge-brownie chip ice cream. You pad into the kitchen and open the freezer only to discover that your spouse polished it off the night before. What do you do? Do you think, "oh well," and go back to bed? Or do you hop in your car, still wearing your bathrobe and slippers, and drive 15 minutes to the 24-hour convenience store to get some of that ice cream and then eat it in the parking lot?

If you picked the latter, you're not alone. Many people with weight issues tend to want immediate rewards:

> **WANT ICE CREAM → EAT ICE CREAM → FEEL BETTER**

If you're trying to lose weight, however, the scenario plays out very differently:

> **WANT ICE CREAM → RESIST ICE CREAM → FEEL FRUSTRATED**

The problem with most diets is that there's no form of immediate gratification. You just have to deprive yourself in order to reach your goals. Yes, reaching your goal weight weeks or months later may ultimately offer more lasting satisfaction, but it comes up short in terms of making you feel good *right this minute!* But it doesn't have to be that way. We have learned that when you're going to be skipping the chunky fudge-brownie chip ice cream, you need to swap that habit with some sort of non-food reinforcement to provide you with a sense of gratification.

PRACTICE USING NON-FOOD REINFORCERS

This program is designed to provide you with a veritable team of non-food reinforcers to help keep you feeling satisfied. These BioModifiers help you make important physiological changes. They're so powerful that by practicing using them, you can eliminate those old bad habits without feeling deprived.

- **Reading this book:** Every time you read a chapter, it reinforces the reasons why you're saying no to the ice cream and staying focused on the greater reward.

- **Doing the DAP:** Doing all the things you need to do to complete your DAP—taking your ketostick reading, weighing yourself, tracking your food intake, planning for obstacles and more—lets you see daily progress and gives you a sense of accomplishment.

- **Reviewing your "My Motivator Cards":** Looking at your "My Motivator Cards" at times when you're craving something very tempting can be a good way to keep your eye on the prize.

- **Looking at your "After" photo:** Envisioning your body the way it will be when you reach your goal—remember, this is a form of episodic future thinking—makes your goal more salient and gives you a more immediate sense of satisfaction.

- **Doing weekly progress reports:** Looking at all the progress you've made can make you feel more confident about your ability to stick with the program.

Access information about coaching and support to help you with your program.

The more practice you put into these habits, the stronger the neural pathways will become and eventually, they will become automatized behaviors that you don't even have to think about. You'll just do them naturally. You may already be doing some of them automatically.

LEAN FOR LIFE-APPROVED FOOD REINFORCERS

We know that non-food reinforcers aren't always going to make up for that bowl of ice cream you really want right now. That's why you can also choose from dozens of delicious Lean for Life and KOT protein snacks that pack all the great flavor you want and still keep you on the path to weight loss.

The Inside Story from Dr. Allouche

DON'T LET OLD HABITS DOG YOU

Have you heard of Pavlov's dogs? Ivan Pavlov, a Russian physiologist, used dogs in one of the most famous scientific trials ever. In the presence of the dogs, Pavlov would ring a bell and then offer food to the dogs. At the outset of the trial, the food would cause the dogs to salivate. After repeated sessions over time, however, simply ringing the bell would cause the dogs to drool. This has become known as a *conditioned response*.

You may not have realized it, but you have likely been the subject of conditioning yourself, only in your case, you're both the scientist doing the conditioning and the "subject" being conditioned. Think about it. When that cupcake shop first opened near your work, you walked over after lunch and got a cupcake for dessert. Now, months later, after visiting the cupcake shop every workday, as soon as you start eating your lunch, you're already thinking about that cupcake you're going to get. Okay, so maybe you don't drool all over your desk like Pavlov's dogs—at least, I hope not!—but you have a conditioned response just the same.

Changing your habits is a matter of *reconditioning*. For example, instead of heading straight to the cupcake shop after lunch, you're going to need to substitute that with something that will reward your brain, such as a 10-minute walk or sitting in the sunshine with a good book while having a cup of delicious hot tea. Over time—remember, it took time to develop your cupcake habit, too—you'll be conditioned to pair lunch with a break that is self-nurturing and healthy.

What you'll eventually discover is that *intentionally* doing something else provides you with something called *intrinsic reinforcement*, which is kind of like giving yourself an internal pat on the back. Researchers agree that the ability to control your actions can lead to the release of serotonin that makes you feel good about yourself and your decision. So whether you're reading, taking a walk, or having a cup of tea instead of devouring that cupcake, you start to like your new healthy habits more and more. All of this adds up to increased motivation to reach your ultimate goal of being Lean for Life.

DAY 28: MENU DAY

A DAY TO LOOK BACK AND LOOK AHEAD

Congratulations! You've reached Day 28! Over the past four weeks, you've faced—and met—many challenges. You've had the opportunity to use new skills in overcoming obstacles. You've learned to be successful at losing weight. You're looking and feeling healthier than you did just four weeks ago. Completing four weeks of this program is a major stepping-stone toward becoming Lean for Life, but it isn't the end of the line. Today, we'll help you determine what your next step will be. However, before you forge ahead onto the next part of your journey, it's a good idea to assess what you've learned so far and to acknowledge how far you've come. That's why today is devoted to both looking back and moving ahead.

REVIEW YOUR 28-DAY JOURNEY

In the past 28 days, you have accomplished so much more than just losing weight. Today is a good day to reflect on your journey so far.

1. **Take a few moments and think about the most important things you've learned.** What have you discovered about the following?

   - Your eating habits.
   - Your physical activity.
   - Your thinking habits.
   - Your brain.
   - Your body.
   - Your gut.

   Then spend some time reflecting on how you can use that information going forward to help you maintain your weight loss.

2. **Make a list of the specific eating strategies, BioModifiers, thought control techniques, exercise recommendations and stress relievers that have proven to be most helpful to you.** Write down the page numbers where these tips are detailed so you can refer back to them often. Or simply flag those pages in this book for easy reference. It's important to remember that the repetition of reading and re-reading these tips will help strengthen the new neural pathways you've developed.

3. **Acknowledge the parts of the program that have been the most challenging or confusing for you.** We know that this program has worked for hundreds of thousands of people, but we also know that most of our patients experience challenges with at least one aspect of it along the way. You're probably no different. What's your biggest challenge? Is it moving more? Curbing cravings? Dealing with stress? Make a commitment to keep working on whatever it is that you find difficult and re-read the sections that cover the things you struggle with. The more times you go through the material, the more likely it is that the behavior will become easier.

4. **Reflect on your rewards.** What positive changes do you notice in your body? In what ways do you look and feel better today compared to 28 days ago? What do you like best about the changes you've made? How have the changes you've made positively impacted the way you feel about yourself and the way you relate to others?

Dr. Stamper Says

THE SIX ESSENTIALS—ESSENTIAL #6: MAINTAIN HEALTHY BEHAVIORS FOR LASTING SUCCESS.

In order to become Lean for Life, you must maintain the healthy behaviors that you've been learning throughout this program. Reaching your ideal lean weight doesn't mean that you've been "cured" or that you can go back to your old eating and thinking habits. The only way to maintain your new lean weight is to maintain the behaviors that got you back to lean. Continue to practice the strategies and techniques you've been learning on this program to increase your success at becoming Lean for Life.

The Inside Story from Dr. Allouche

THE "LEANIFICATION" OF YOUR BRAIN, BODY AND GUT

If you've been following this program carefully for the past 28 days, one quick glance in the mirror is all you need to know that your body's gotten leaner on the outside, but what you can't see with your own two eyes is that it's gotten leaner on the inside, too. In many ways, your brain, body and gut have undergone dramatic transformations that have allowed them to start cooperating and communicating effectively again. In essence, you've realigned these three "neighbors" so they are now working for you to help you maintain your leaner physique. Let's take a peek inside so you can see for yourself.

- **Reward system reset.** Remember that angry alligator in your brain–your reptilian brain–that would demand the chips, chocolate, cheesecake and cheeseburgers that contributed to your weight problems? By following this program, you've helped tame that alligator and muted those demands. This doesn't mean you won't ever crave anything again, but your reward system has become sensitized to another type of reward. Your brain is now releasing dopamine when you do something healthy for yourself rather than giving you a squirt of the feel-good chemical only when you're indulging in the foods that made you unhappy with your weight.

- **Satiety and hunger signals strengthened.** Your appetite hormone signals have become regulated so you are more in touch with signs of true hunger as well as feelings of satiety that encourage you to stop eating when you're pleasantly full.

- **Smaller, friendlier fat cells.** By now, your fat cells have shrunk in size and are less likely to be pumping out the harmful substances, such as interleukin-6 and TNF-alpha, that lead to inflammation throughout your body and even in parts of your brain. If you've already reached your ideal lean weight, your fat cells are now secreting friendlier chemicals, such as leptin, that help reduce hunger and increase insulin sensitivity. Your body's leptin receptors have been sensitized to increase the leptin's ability to work more effectively. Dangerous intra-abdominal fat and intramuscular fat have subsided, reducing your risk for disease and optimizing metabolism.

- **Insulin sensitivity boosted.** After 28 days of eating the foods on this program, you've boosted your body's sensitivity to insulin action. In part, this is due to a sort of reawakening of your body's insulin receptors. This means insulin is better able to do its job of clearing glucose from the bloodstream and ushering it where it needs to go. With less insulin circulating aimlessly in the body, it's easier to maintain weight loss.

- **Inflammation cooled.** By eating the anti-inflammatory foods on this program and practicing the inflammation-fighting BioModifiers, you've cooled the flame within. Reducing inflammation lowers your risk for disease and increases your ability to keep weight off.

- **Liver "leanified."** Because your fat cells are no longer overstuffed, the fat stores in your liver may be decreasing. This reduces the incidence of fatty liver disease and allows the liver to get back to its vital functions in digestion, metabolism and blood sugar regulation.

- **Good news for the gut.** By eating the recommended foods on this program that nourish the beneficial bugs in your gut and by reducing your consumption of the foods that fuel harmful bacteria, you've begun rebalancing your gut microflora. Learning to move more and stress less has also helped reduce the number of troublemaking bugs in your gut. Because of this, your gut is less likely to cause digestive problems or contribute to uncontrollable cravings, and it is more likely to calm cravings, reduce appetite and help you keep your weight down.

- **Better pH balance.** By now, your body is less acidic, which means it doesn't have to work so hard to fight off acidic toxins; instead, it can focus its attention on other processes, such as metabolism. Higher metabolism means you can eat more without gaining weight.

GETTING READY FOR THE NEXT STEP—
WHERE DO YOU GO FROM HERE?

Where do you go next on your journey to becoming Lean for Life? It depends. Determine which of the following statements best fits your current status to discover your next step.

☐ **I have already reached my ideal lean weight.**

Yay! If you've reached your lean weight, you may be tempted to say "Hooray!" and be done with the whole thing. Not so fast! Remember, this program is called Lean for Life not "lean for a month." It's time to move on to the next step, Metabolic Adjustment, starting tomorrow. The following chapter details everything you need to know about this vital 14-day portion of the program that is essential for maintaining weight loss.

☐ **I have more weight to lose and want to continue actively losing weight.**

Many of our patients are so excited about their weight loss after four weeks that they don't want anything to interrupt it. If you're actively losing weight and want to keep your progress going strong, simply go back to Day 1 and repeat the four-week program. Take note: You may only repeat the four-week program once for a total of eight weeks of Rapid Weight Loss before proceeding to the Metabolic Adjustment phase. If you have completed eight weeks of active weight loss and still have more weight to lose, proceed to the Metabolic Adjustment phase for two weeks then repeat the Rapid Weight Loss phase by going back to Day 1.

☐ **I have more weight to lose but would like to take a temporary break from active weight loss.**

You can take a temporary break from active weight loss by moving on to Metabolic Adjustment, which is described in the following chapter. When you are ready to start losing weight again, go back to Day 1 and repeat the 4-week Rapid Weight Loss phase to re-ignite weight loss.

You can continue cycling from the four-week Rapid Weight Loss phase to the Metabolic Adjustment phase as many times as it takes to reach your lean weight goal.

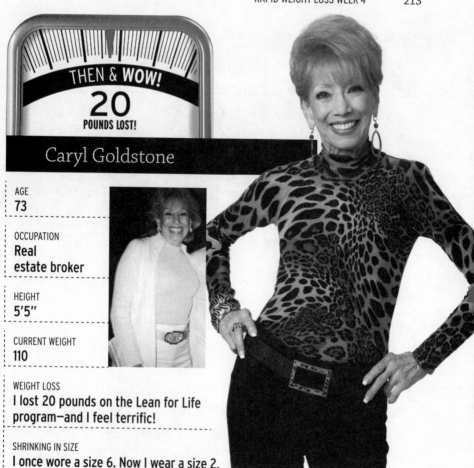

THEN & **WOW!**

20
POUNDS LOST!

Caryl Goldstone

AGE
73

OCCUPATION
Real estate broker

HEIGHT
5'5"

CURRENT WEIGHT
110

WEIGHT LOSS
I lost 20 pounds on the Lean for Life program—and I feel terrific!

SHRINKING IN SIZE
I once wore a size 6. Now I wear a size 2.

Thanks to the Lean for Life program, I feel better than I have in a very long time. I'm living proof that it's never too late to improve your health and to look and feel your best!

THE WOW FACTOR: I volunteer in the emergency room of a major Los Angeles hospital. It's so busy there that people rarely have time to even nod to each other. One day after I lost weight, I went to the hospital dressed for dinner to pick up a friend. A young doctor whom I had not seen for some time saw me, stopped in his tracks and said, "Wow, Caryl, you look amazing!" When people notice the progress you've made, it feels incredible!

PLATEAU PERSISTENCE: Early in my program, I hit a plateau. Even though I was following the program 100 percent, I didn't lose a pound for an entire

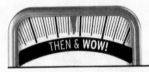

week. After the third day of no weight loss, I even checked the batteries in my bathroom scale. Fortunately, my desire to lose weight was greater than my frustration. I trusted the program enough to know I would break through the plateau, and I did! When the scale finally showed a 3-pound weight loss in two days, I was totally energized. I knew my persistence had paid off.

BYE-BYE BORING: I always thought that in order to lose weight, I had to eat boring, flavorless food. This program has shown me how to enjoy delicious, real food I can buy in grocery stores or order in restaurants. Best of all, I didn't feel deprived while I was losing weight.

PORTION POWER: I often used to eat until I felt full. The program has really taught me portion control. I can't remember the last time I ate an entire portion at a restaurant. I always leave at least half of my meal, and I rarely order desserts.

TODAY'S THE DAY: I work with women in their 30s and 40s who tell me they would love to have my figure—and my energy—when they're my age. I tell them all about Lean for Life and ask them, "What are you waiting for?" There's no better day than today to begin living the life you want.

IT'S YOUR CHOICE: Having been a hospital volunteer for 17 years, I've often noticed that many of the overweight or obese patients also have heart disease, type 2 diabetes and other health complications. There is no doubt in my mind there is a direct connection between our diets and our longevity. There is so much in life we can't control, but we can make better choices every day. At 73, I'm eating better and moving more. As a result, life is wonderful!

METABOLIC ADJUSTMENT:

THE KEY TO EATING MORE WITHOUT GAINING WEIGHT

8

Did you know that following a period of carbohydrate restriction, reverting immediately back to your old eating habits can result in gaining 5 to 10 pounds of water weight in a matter of days? We've seen it happen with patients who lose weight on Rapid Weight Loss but then stray from the program and opt *not* to follow the prescribed guidelines for the all-important Metabolic Adjustment phase. New science confirms that you can prevent rebound weight gain by increasing carbohydrate consumption *gradually* over time. This is exactly what you'll be doing during Metabolic Adjustment, and it is how hundreds of thousands of Lean for Lifers have already learned how to eat more without gaining weight following Rapid Weight Loss. In this chapter, we'll give you everything you need to know so you can start enjoying more food and more carbs without putting on the pounds.

WHAT IS METABOLIC ADJUSTMENT?

Metabolic Adjustment is a vital phase that lasts a *minimum* of 14 days and is essential to becoming Lean for Life. During this period, you'll begin gradually eating more food and more carbohydrates, making additions according to a specific schedule. You'll also continue the success strategies you've learned throughout Rapid Weight Loss—maintaining your DAP (you'll find special

DAP forms for each level of Metabolic Adjustment in Appendix A), engaging in physical activity, using the mental training techniques you find most helpful and more. What you won't be doing is intentionally losing weight.

Important! The goal of Metabolic Adjustment is not to lose weight, but rather to gradually increase your food and carbohydrate intake without gaining weight.

This concept is difficult for many of our patients to accept, which is why we want you to be prepared for it. Metabolic Adjustment is straightforward and easy to follow, but it is the part of the program during which our patients are most likely to trip up and interrupt their success. We find that the inner sabotage agent denial can be especially dangerous during this portion of the program. From our patients we hear things like:

- "I don't want to stop losing weight so I'm not going to do Metabolic Adjustment."

- "I just needed help losing weight. Now that I have, I don't need to do Metabolic Adjustment because I know how to maintain my weight."

- "I really pigged out last night, so I'm not going to weigh myself today. I don't want to know if I've gained weight because that would just discourage me."

- "I don't really have to follow the Metabolic Adjustment menus. After all, I'm not trying to stay in ketosis."

Because we have found that denial can derail your progress here, we urge you to revisit Day 6 for a refresher on how to mute this inner sabotage agent.

Many of our patients, especially those who have yet to reach their ideal lean weight, resist doing this phase of the program. And it's easy to understand why. If your ultimate goal is to lose more weight, you don't want to stall your progress. And you may be worried that at the end of Metabolic Adjustment, you won't be able to re-ignite the fat-burning fire. Wrong! Following this portion of the program actually makes it easier to kick-start weight loss. If you fail to complete this part of the program, however, you may soon find it difficult or even impossible to lose weight. You may manage to shed a few extra bonus pounds, but they'll come off much more slowly due to metabolic adaptation and you'll likely regain those pounds—and more.

If you have already reached your ideal lean weight, you may find yourself resisting Metabolic Adjustment for other reasons. You may think you've crossed the finish line and can cross "lose weight" off your to-do list forever. Not so fast. When you fail to adjust your metabolism and start increasing your calorie intake without guidance, you're likely to regain weight rapidly because your body hasn't had a chance to adjust to the intake of extra fuel. Even if you substitute foods on the Metabolic Adjustment menus for others that contain the same number of calories, you run the risk of decreasing your muscle mass and increasing your body fat, which is the opposite of your goal to get leaner.

We cannot stress enough how important it is for you to approach this step in the program with as much enthusiasm as you have devoted to the past four weeks. Don't worry—we'll help you get through it with flying colors.

THE BENEFITS OF METABOLIC ADJUSTMENT

To help you understand why the Metabolic Adjustment step is so critical for maintaining weight loss, let's look at the benefits it provides. During Metabolic Adjustment, your body will:

- Adjust to the significant reduction in body fat it has experienced, so you can eat more calories *without gaining back any of the fat you lost.*

- Adjust your body chemistry back to a state in which you're no longer in ketosis and you are able to eat more carbohydrates again *without gaining weight.*

- Adjust your metabolic rate upwards so that you're burning more calories and are able to eat more food *without gaining weight.*

- Adjust—or at least begin the physiological process of adjusting—your setpoint to your new lower weight so you can enjoy eating enough so you're not hungry *without gaining weight.*

- Adjust your digestion process to restore the normal physiological pattern of using carbs and fat for fuel *without storing carbs and fat as fat.*

WHY IS IT SO IMPORTANT TO ADJUST YOUR METABOLISM?

Whenever your body is forced to function on a reduced number of calories, as it has been doing over the past 28 days, it eventually adapts and trains itself to get by on whatever calories it's getting—*without losing weight.* You can thank, or rather blame, the body's built-in survival mechanism known as "metabolic adaptation" for this. It's your body's way of protecting you from starvation.

Metabolic adaptation was a real lifesaver for our ancestors—remember Caveman Krunk and Cavewoman Gurk from Day 5 who sometimes had to survive for days, weeks or even months when food was scarce? This natural process helped keep them from wasting away. But when you're actively trying to get leaner, metabolic adaptation can stall weight loss despite your best efforts. And that can be so frustrating. We've found that it's one of the main reasons why so many people give up their weight-loss efforts and revert back to their old habits. Don't let this happen to you!

You're standing at a very important crossroads in your journey to becoming Lean for Life, and what you do during Metabolic Adjustment can either enhance your ability to be successful or begin to undo all the hard work you've put in so far. It's up to you.

INSTRUCTIONS FOR METABOLIC ADJUSTMENT

Remember, Metabolic Adjustment lasts a *minimum* of 14 days. It's okay if it takes you longer than two weeks to complete, as this phase is individualized to you and your unique physiology. Metabolic Adjustment is divided into three levels. With each level, gradually increase the amount of food you are consuming according to the following guidelines. Remember, the foods you'll be eating are identical to those in Rapid Weight Loss; it is only the *portion sizes* that change. Keep eating three meals and three high PER protein snacks per day and continue doing one Protein Day per week. See "Metabolic Adjustment Menu Plans" for specific menu guidelines.

- **Day 1 (Protein Day):** Follow the guidelines for Protein Days in Rapid Weight Loss.

- **Level 1 (Days 2–3):** Increase to 2 proteins at breakfast and 1½ proteins at both lunch and dinner. Also increase to 1½ fruits or grains at breakfast.

- **Level 2 (Days 4–7):** Increase to 2 proteins at both lunch and dinner.

- **Day 8 (Protein Day):** Follow the guidelines for Protein Days in Rapid Weight Loss.

- **Level 3 (Days 9–14):** Add 1 grain to both lunch and dinner.

METABOLIC ADJUSTMENT MENU PLANS

DAY 1	LEVEL 1	LEVEL 2	DAY 8	LEVEL 3
Protein Day	(Days 2-3)	(Days 4-7)	Protein Day	(Days 9-14)

BREAKFAST

	LEVEL 1	LEVEL 2		LEVEL 3
	2 Proteins	2 Proteins		2 Proteins
	1½ Fruit or Grain	1½ Fruit or Grain		1½ Fruit or Grain
	1 Beverage	1 Beverage		1 Beverage

PROTEIN SNACK

LUNCH

	LEVEL 1	LEVEL 2		LEVEL 3
	1½ Proteins	2 Proteins		2 Proteins
	1 Vegetable	1 Vegetable		1 Vegetable
	Lettuce (unlimited)	Lettuce (unlimited)		Lettuce (unlimited)
	1 Fruit	1 Fruit		1 Fruit
	1 Beverage	1 Beverage		1 Beverage
	2 Misc	2 Misc		2 Misc
				1 Grain

PROTEIN SNACK

DINNER

	LEVEL 1	LEVEL 2		LEVEL 3
	1½ Proteins	2 Proteins		2 Proteins
	1 Vegetable	1 Vegetable		1 Vegetable
	Lettuce (unlimited)	Lettuce (unlimited)		Lettuce (unlimited)
	1 Fruit	1 Fruit		1 Fruit
	1 Beverage	1 Beverage		1 Beverage
	2 Misc	2 Misc		2 Misc
				1 Grain

WATCH OUT FOR THE 1½-POUND ALARM

During Metabolic Adjustment, the goal is to stay within 1½ pounds of your new lower weight. If you ever experience a weight gain of 1½ pounds or more, think of it as an alarm going off and take immediate action by making the rest of your meals that day be protein meals rather than eating the menu foods indicated for that day. The extra weight should be gone by the next morning. If you really overindulged, you may need to continue eating protein meals for more than one day. *Do not proceed to the next level until you have increased quantities as directed and maintained your weight within 1½ pounds* (based on your weight at the beginning of each level). Remember, it's okay if it takes you longer than 14 days to complete Metabolic Adjustment.

What makes 1½ pounds the magic number? Everybody's body weight fluctuates to some degree—you're ½ pound up one day and down ½ pound the next. It's adding weight day after day that is cause for concern. The 1½-pound alarm establishes a clear guideline that will help you prevent a minor fluctuation from becoming a major weight gain. This is why it is so important for you to continue weighing yourself every morning during Metabolic Adjustment.

We have pinpointed the three most common reasons why people struggle with weight gain during Metabolic Adjustment:

- Eating too much of the approved foods on the "Lean Foods" lists.

- Eating foods that are not on the approved "Lean Foods" lists.

- Not getting enough physical activity.

To find out what's holding you up, review your DAP for clues. Have you been forgetting to write down *everything* you eat and drink? Have you been overdoing it on your portion sizes? Have you been indulging in foods that aren't on the menu? Have you been skipping your walks or workouts? As you learned during Rapid Weight Loss, being aware of your habits is the first step to changing them so you can get back on track.

12 LEAN HABITS FOR SUCCESS ON METABOLIC ADJUSTMENT

1. Weigh yourself each morning.
2. Do one Protein Day each week.

3. Eat three meals a day.

4. Eat two high PER protein snacks a day.

5. Stick to the approved Lean Foods.

6. Drink at least 80 ounces of water or other calorie-free fluid every day.

7. Take your vitamins and supplements.

8. Keep moving more and monitoring your steps.

9. Continue practicing relaxation techniques.

10. Maintain your DAP.

11. Continue your brain training techniques.

12. Maintain your motivation.

Once you've completed this phase, you'll have a decision to make. You can either repeat Rapid Weight Loss to continue losing weight or, if you've reached your ideal lean weight, you can advance to the next step of the program: Metabolic Equilibrium.

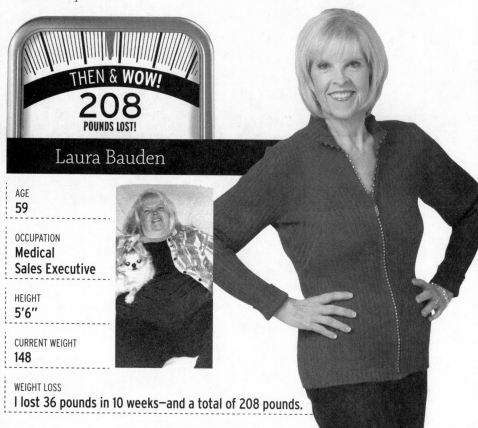

THEN & **WOW!**

208

POUNDS LOST!

Laura Bauden

AGE
59

OCCUPATION
Medical Sales Executive

HEIGHT
5'6"

CURRENT WEIGHT
148

WEIGHT LOSS
I lost 36 pounds in 10 weeks—and a total of 208 pounds.

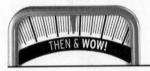

SIZE DOES MATTER
I used to wear a size 28/30. Now I wear a size 8.

BMI
My BMI dropped from 56 (obese) to 24 (normal).

Before I did the Lean for Life program, my body was giving out, and I was giving up. I weighed 356 pounds and was taking medication for high cholesterol, high blood pressure and type 2 diabetes. Not anymore!

EMBRACE THE PROCESS: I understand the temptation to skip Metabolic Adjustment. After all, it's human nature to want more of a good thing. When I came to the end of my first Lean for Life Rapid Weight Loss phase, I was losing weight so rapidly that I just wanted to continue losing. I didn't want to break my stride and mess with my momentum. But once I understood that the goal of Metabolic Adjustment was to gradually help my body adapt to eating more food and more carbs without gaining weight, I knew I needed to relax, stop resisting and just follow the program as it was created. I felt like the program had earned my trust—and I knew from experience that doing things my way didn't work. If it did, I wouldn't have been 200 pounds overweight.

MY "AFTER" PHOTO COME TRUE: I lived 40 years as a "Before" photo. When I look at photos of myself today, I look younger—and healthier— than I did 20 years ago. I'm loving it!

MYSTERY WOMAN: I get a kick out of it when people I haven't seen in a while don't recognize me. I've walked up to people I've known for years and said hello, and it's obvious they have no clue who I am. When they realize it's me, the first thing they say is: "You look so great!" I have to admit that's something I never get tired of hearing.

METABOLIC EQUILIBRIUM:
STAYING LEAN FOR LIFE

9

Welcome to the first day of the rest of your lean life! In this chapter, we'll introduce you to the final phase for *staying* Lean for Life—Metabolic Equilibrium—and we'll give you tools to make it work for you.

WHAT IS METABOLIC EQUILIBRIUM?

Metabolic Equilibrium is a lifestyle program intended to keep you Lean for Life. You can think of this phase as "preventive maintenance." If you continue to make healthy choices as you've learned to do so far in this program, you can prevent weight regain!

During this phase, you'll be eating an even wider variety of foods to see the changes you've been making to your brain, body and gut in action! Even though you get to continue increasing the amount of food you're eating on a daily basis during Metabolic Equilibrium, you may find this cycle to be challenging. Now that you've reached this phase, you may no longer feel the sense of urgency to comply with a structured program. You may have "lost steam" after weeks of intense focus on changing your habits. You may feel like you're "cured" and that your brain and body have been reset and will do everything for you now. You may feel like you've "finished" the program and can go back to your old habits. Wrong!

Although your biochemistry has been changed for the better, and your brain, body and gut are working to help keep you at your new lean weight, you still need to maintain focus. That's exactly what this final phase is designed to help you do.

If you want to maintain your new lean weight, you must maintain the behavior changes that made it happen.

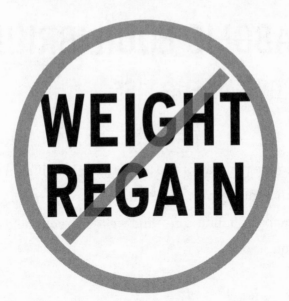

Metabolic Equilibrium is the key to preventing weight regain.

STABILIZE AT YOUR NEW LEAN WEIGHT

Your goal during Metabolic Equilibrium is simple and specific—stabilize at your new lean weight so you will be able to maintain it for life. It typically takes at least 3 to 12 months to stabilize your weight. How will you know when you've done it? By eating a "test meal," a big evening meal consisting of larger portions of the foods you've become accustomed to eating on this program. How large of a meal do we mean? Not quite as big as a Thanksgiving feast, but if you go to a chain restaurant, order a dinner meal, and clean your plate, that should be big enough. The next morning, hop on the scale.

- **For smaller women, if your weight is within 1½ pounds of your lean weight, or within 3 pounds for taller women and men:** Pat yourself on the back because your weight has stabilized.

- **For smaller women, if you've gained more than 1½ pounds, or for taller women and men if you're more than 3 pounds over your lean weight:** This indicates that your weight still hasn't stabilized. In this case, revert to having a protein meal for your evening meals until you get back down to your lean weight. After you've accomplished that, your goal is to stay within 3 pounds of your lean weight for another three to four weeks.

Then try again with another test meal. Keep repeating this process until you can eat the test meal without gaining weight.

When you've achieved stabilization at your lean weight, you'll be able to consume greater quantities of food and carbohydrates—*within reason*—without putting on extra pounds. This doesn't mean you'll be able to resume your old eating habits. You will, however, be able to eat more generous amounts of healthy foods and even splurge occasionally and still stay Lean for Life.

"HOW MUCH CAN I EAT?"

The quantity of food you'll be able to eat without gaining weight depends on a number of factors, including your gender, current weight and activity level. For example, an inactive 140-pound woman typically needs only 10–12 calories per pound of body weight to maintain her weight—somewhere in the neighborhood of 1,400 to 1,680 calories. An active 190-pound man, on the other hand, may be able to consume 14 to 16 calories per pound of body weight—2,660 to 3,040 calories—without gaining weight. The "How Much Can I Eat" chart in Appendix G will help you estimate how many calories your body needs to maintain your present weight. It will also help you plan meals to ensure you achieve a healthy balance of macronutrients.

On this portion of the program, it's not just the *quantity* of the food you eat that matters, it's the percentages of each food group. As a rule, your daily intake should consist of 45 percent carbohydrates, 25 percent protein and 30 percent fat. To maximize your results, you may restrict your fat intake to less than 30 percent—about 35 to 45 grams for women, and 45 to 60 grams for men. The calories you "save" can then be used for either more protein or more healthy complex carbs. To see how your daily meals would shape up, see the "Metabolic Equilibrium Menu Plan" on page 226.

METABOLIC EQUILIBRIUM MENU PLAN

BREAKFAST

Protein

Fruit

Grain

Beverage

MID-MORNING SNACK (OPTIONAL)

High PER protein snack

LUNCH

Protein

Vegetable (unlimited)

Lettuce or greens

Grain

Fruit

Misc

Beverage

MID-AFTERNOON SNACK

High PER protein snack

DINNER

Protein

Vegetable (unlimited)

Lettuce or greens

Grain

Fruit

Misc

Beverage

METABOLIC EQUILIBRIUM MENU PLAN

EVENING SNACK (OPTIONAL)

High PER protein snack

WATCH OUT FOR THE 3-POUND ALARM

Remember the 1½-pound alarm you learned about during Metabolic Adjustment? During Metabolic Equilibrium, it's a 3-pound alarm. If you ever gain more than 3 pounds over your lean weight or your Rapid Weight Loss ending weight, it should set off a mental alarm in your brain, alerting you that it's time to take action. As you did during Metabolic Adjustment, make your next meal a protein meal and continue having protein meals until you get back to your lean weight.

Why should you set your mental alarm for 3 pounds? We have found that if our patients gain more than 3 pounds, it means they have begun to stray from their lean behaviors and have fallen back into some old patterns. To prevent those old habits from undoing all the rewiring of your brain circuits you have accomplished while on this program, it is absolutely critical to put a halt to them quickly. Staying within 3 pounds of your lean weight ensures that you are sticking with the habits that helped you become lean.

6 HABITS OF SUCCESSFUL LEAN FOR LIFERS

What makes some people such successful Lean for Lifers? Over the years, our clinical staff has identified the following six habits that successful maintainers share. Adopt these habits and you'll ensure your status among the Lean for Life club!

1. **Successful Lean for Lifers continue to make the eating habits they've learned and the approved Lean Foods the mainstays of their diet.** Continue doing a Protein Day each week, eating three meals and three protein snacks a day, and drinking at least 80 ounces of calorie-free fluids each day. Stick with it! You've also retrained your brain and body to enjoy the healthy foods that leanify your body, satisfy

your cravings and help keep you feeling full. Now is no time to go back to regularly eating the foods that messed up your metabolism, hijacked your reward system and increased your appetite. As long as you're staying within 3 pounds of your lean weight, it's okay to splurge *occasionally* on something that isn't on the Lean Foods list. Just watch your portion sizes and incorporate the better eating tools you've learned. *Weigh yourself each morning to make sure the 3-pound alarm isn't blaring.*

2. **Successful Lean for Lifers continue to practice the basics of the program.** Continue putting the strategies you've learned into action during Metabolic Equilibrium, and you'll continue to be successful, too. In particular, continue weighing yourself daily, maintaining your DAP (see the special "DAP for Metabolic Equilibrium" in Appendix A), practicing your mental training techniques and using the stress-less strategies.

3. **Successful Lean for Lifers intentionally develop and maintain their self-image as a lean person.** Use positive affirmations to reinforce your new identity and use the mental training techniques you've learned to think, act and react like a lean person.

4. **Successful Lean for Lifers are physically active.** Some people find that 30 minutes of moderate exercise a day isn't enough to maintain their lean weight, so they add more physical activity throughout their day.

5. **Successful Lean for Lifers plan ahead for high-risk situations.** Use the tools and strategies in this book to come up with a plan to deal with challenging situations *before* they happen.

6. **Successful Lean for Lifers develop and maintain a support system.** This is especially important during the first 12 months of Metabolic Equilibrium. You can get support in a variety of ways. Lean on friends and family, enroll in one of our clinics or online programs, sign up for our phone coaching or take advantage of all the support available on the Lean for Life website. The book you are holding in your hands is another form of support. *The New Lean for Life* is not intended to be read once and then placed forever on the bookshelf. It is one of the most powerful support tools you have at your disposal and should be read and re-read frequently. Wherever you turn for support, make a point to stay connected with the people and things that encourage your efforts to remain Lean for Life.

STAYING LEAN FOR LIFE CHECKLIST

Throughout this book, you've discovered how to use the most up-to-date scientific findings, the latest weight-loss tools, and the most impactful mental training techniques to outsmart your biology and get your brain, body and gut working for you. With your "BBG gang" on your side, you've been shrinking your fat cells and making it easier than ever to achieve your goal of becoming Lean for Life. As you continue on your journey, put the following checklist into practice to keep your brain, body and gut working for you so you can remain Lean for Life.

☐ Weigh yourself every day. If your weight is up 3 pounds, make your next meal a protein meal.

☐ Move more.

☐ Take advantage of high PER protein foods that stave off hunger and increase satiety.

☐ Continue to make low-glycemic foods the foundation of your meals. Beware of hidden sugars, especially HFCS, in processed foods.

☐ Increase your intake of omega-3 fatty acids and reduce your intake of omega-6 fatty acids.

☐ Feed your good gut bacteria with healthy fiber, and don't fuel harmful bacteria with sugars and refined carbs.

☐ Stress less to reduce cravings and mindless eating.

☐ Cook at home as often as possible; eat meals at the table without distractions from the TV, cell phone or newspaper; take at least 20 minutes to finish eating.

☐ Limit alcohol consumption.

☐ Continue to learn about food and your body in the ongoing process of becoming Lean for Life.

And if you find yourself gaining weight and slipping back into old habits that caused you to gain weight in the first place, we're here to help! You can always get back on the path to becoming Lean for Life. It's as simple as opening the book and starting again at Day 1. We wish you a long and healthy life!

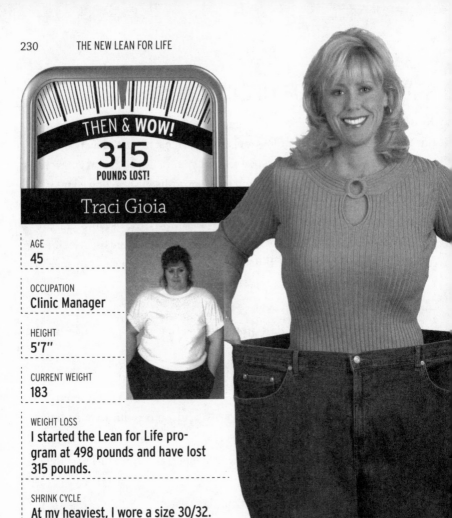

THEN & WOW!

315
POUNDS LOST!

Traci Gioia

AGE
45

OCCUPATION
Clinic Manager

HEIGHT
5'7"

CURRENT WEIGHT
183

WEIGHT LOSS
I started the Lean for Life program at 498 pounds and have lost 315 pounds.

SHRINK CYCLE
At my heaviest, I wore a size 30/32. Now I wear a size 8.

At 498 pounds, I felt like I was dying a little every day. Today, I'm very alive, very active and very grateful! The Lean for Life program literally gave me my life back.

BEEN THERE, DONE THAT: I'd tried everything from diet plans to diet pills. Nothing ever worked for me—until I did the Lean for Life program.

THE BIG DIFFERENCE: For me, the program wasn't about deprivation or what I couldn't eat. It was about learning to eat in healthier ways and overcoming all of the bad habits that had literally been weighing me down.

PLAN OF ACTION: The Lean for Life program really taught me the value of being prepared and always planning ahead. I take my lunch to work every day, for example, because it allows me to control what and how much

I eat. If I'm going out to dinner with friends, I'll check out the restaurant's website to make sure they offer some healthy selections.

GOING THE DISTANCE: I often tell people that the program isn't about changing your diet as much as it is about changing your life. What I know from maintaining a 315-pound weight loss for nearly 11 years is that when you continue doing what has worked for you, you will continue to enjoy success. You can't revert back to old habits and expect your results to last.

MOVING MORE AND LIKING IT: At 498 pounds, just walking from my desk to the copier was a challenge. My back and knees hurt all the time, and I was always out of breath. Today, I work out or run two hours a day, seven days a week. If I'm not at the gym, I'm walking or running or playing softball. I don't do it because I have to—I do it because I enjoy it.

ROLE MODEL: It feels so amazing when people tell me how much I've inspired them. My story has been featured in *People* magazine, on the cover of two national women's magazines, and on several local and national TV shows. I love sharing my story because I know there are people who will look at what I've accomplished and think to themselves, *If she did it, maybe I can, too*. I'm living proof that you can!

ACKNOWLEDGMENTS

CYNTHIA STAMPER GRAFF

I am grateful to so many people who helped make this book a reality. "Merci beaucoup" to my co-author Réginald Allouche, M.D., whose fascinating research coupled with his charming wit and unbridled passion for the science of weight loss have added a special dimension to *Lean for Life*. Kudos to Frances Sharpe, our wonderful writing partner, for making both of us look good on paper. I will always cherish the excitement and laughter as we collaborated, like when we first visualized the incredible journey of a piece of pizza!

Thank you to the hard-working, caring, and compassionate Team Lindora for sharing the clinical experience, patient stories, and "secrets" that have made the Lean For Life program so successful. I am filled with pride to call you colleagues. A special nod goes to the following remarkable individuals who have been with me for more than 10 years: Jamie Allen, Al Andres, Claudia Ayala, Clare Barker, Olivia Beltz, Flo Buchanan, Suzanne Burrows, Charmaine Calderon, Monica Carroll, Maria Castro, Lyliane Cheneau, Cynthia Coccia, Janet Coleman, Daphne Collom, Shannon Compton, Anne Marie Coppen, Jayme Davidson, Leslie De La Flor, Cindy Dell Orfano, JoAnn Deller, Cynthia Encinas, Lisa Gause, Christine Gil, Ann Gillespie, Danielle Gray, Joyce Hefner, Linda Hughes, Patricia Iacono, Deborah Jones, Vicki Kimura, Holly LaFata, Angela Major, Paola Martinez, Nayra Merchain, Kim Meyer, Monica Penticoff, Shirley Prather, Christina Quarles, Mike Quinn, Debbie Riley, Tiffany Robertson, Janet Schmitt, Lena Sherman, Melanie Smith, Deborah Sozzani, Dollie Tenorio, Sherrie Theckston, Aracelie Tucker, Joe Walton, Meg Whittington, Elaine Wilt and Mark Wisniewski. And Peter Vash, M.D., I so appreciate all the years together.

I would like to acknowledge the following incredible go-getters who make my "day job" so much easier: Marilyn Platfoot, Lori Fish, Leslie Kipnis, Stephanie Bridson, Pat Dobremsyl, Janette Bennett, Kathy Ayres, Dustin Chaney and Ryan Smaligo; Aethra Gervase, Holly Stamper and Juli So for the work you do with Rite Aid; and Jerry Holderman, who is still my "go to" guy after 20 years! Frank Groff and Roger Riddell, you have worked magic to get our message out there.

And to Dr. George Blackburn, I thank you for the years of friendship and the special access you've given me to you and your incredible scientific network.

I'm beyond grateful to our impressive literary agent Yfat Reiss Gendell, not only for her sharp insights, but also for introducing us to the incredible team at Harlequin. I'm so thankful to have had the good fortune to entrust this book to such a talented and thoughtful editor, Sarah Pelz. You have been a delight to work with. Thank you for your belief in *Lean for Life*.

To my family, words are barely adequate to express my love and gratitude. I hope you see your collective fingerprints throughout this book. Steve and Bernie Stamper, thank you for all the years of working together. Kitty, you are always so thoughtful. My strong and smart mother, Nell, thank you for your constant encouragement. My beautiful daughter, Ali, who aspires to become a physician to carry on our family tradition, I am so proud of you. And special thanks to Dr. Marshall Stamper, my father, my mentor, my hero, whose legendary commitment to his patients spawned the Lean For Life revolution.

I must recognize the hundreds of thousands of people who have already put their trust in this program. Seeing you lose weight, get healthier and become Lean for Life with this program is my greatest joy.

RÉGINALD ALLOUCHE, M.D.

First of all, I would like to thank my co-author, Cynthia Stamper Graff, and our "Franco-American alliance," which allowed this book to come to fruition. We share the same vision and are both dedicated to helping people not only reach their weight goals but also become healthier inside and out. I must also acknowledge Dr. Marshall Stamper, a true pioneer in the field. May I have the good fortune to follow in your footsteps by continuing to build on your groundbreaking work. I have a debt of gratitude to our writing partner Frances Sharpe, who has two indispensable qualities—she understands science like a scientist and she understands French. This helped a lot! In addition, I feel it is my duty to recognize the following scientific researchers and collaborators whose tireless work continues to inspire me every day:

- Dr. Florence Massiera, my longtime research collaborator.
- Max Lafontan, Ph.D., and Gérard Ailhaud, Ph.D., for their groundbreaking work in the area of fat cell metabolism.

- Gilles Mithieux, Ph.D., for his discoveries of intestinal neoglucogenesis and peptide action on satiety.

- Karine Clément Ph.D., for our joint efforts in researching gut microflora and for our studies appearing in the *American Journal of Clinical Nutrition and Nature* in 2013.

- Dr. Serge Luquet for collaborating with me in researching the good soluble fibers for our gut microflora.

- Dr. Serge Ahmed for enlightening me on sugar addiction.

I am so appreciative of the entire KOT team in Paris, who do their very best every day to produce this new generation of French gourmet diet food that has been helping so many people for more than 15 years. To our brilliant literary agent, Yfat Reiss Gendell, your support and guidance throughout the publishing process has been invaluable. I am eternally grateful to our amazing editor, Sarah Pelz, and to the entire team at Harlequin. It's been such an honor working with you.

Of course, I am particularly indebted to my wife, Laurence, my daughters, Elsa and Mahaut, and my stepson, David, for supporting me during the writing of this book even when it meant taking time away from my family. My parents, brother, and sister were the first fans of this book and continue to encourage my efforts. I am thankful to be continually inspired by my late grandmother, Anna Franco. And finally, my most heartfelt thoughts go to my late father, Isaac Allouche.

APPENDIX A

DO THE DAP

As you've learned, the Daily Action Plan (DAP) is a simple daily record that will be your constant companion as you learn to eat better, move more and stress less. It is critical to your success. Here you'll find a sample completed DAP for a Rapid Weight Loss Menu Day as well as blank DAPs for every phase of the program. Remember, you can also find these forms online (leanforlife.com).

View DAP forms.

DAP FOR MENU DAYS–SAMPLE

Lean for Life!®

DAILY ACTION PLAN

Week __2__ Day __11__ Date __3/5__

Time		Serving Size	Carbs (grams)
7:00	**Breakfast**		
	Protein egg	1	1
	Fruit or Grain		
	whole	1 slice	15
	wheat toast		
	Beverage coffee	8 oz.	0
10:30	**Snack** low-fat cheese	2 oz.	2
12:30	**Lunch**		
	Protein canned tuna	2½ oz.	0
	Vegetable tomato	1 small	5
	Lettuce	2 cups	3
	Fruit strawberries	1 cup	11
	Beverage water	8 oz.	0
	Miscellaneous		
	fat-free salad dressing	1 tsp.	2
3:30	**Snack** protein bar	1	10
6:15	**Dinner**		
	Protein chicken breast	3½ oz.	0
	Vegetable asparagus	1 cup	8
	Lettuce	2 cups	3
	Fruit tangerine	1 small	9
	Beverage water	30 oz.	0
	Miscellaneous		
	fat-free salad dressing	1 tsp.	2
8:45	**Snack** wildberry passion drink	8 oz.	3
		TOTAL	74

Keto Reading   Moderate

Weight   168

Vitamin   2 AM   2 PM

Water   8, 30, 8, 30, 10, 8 = 94 oz.

Activities/Duration:

30 minute walk, 20 leg lifts and take stairs at work

 # Pedometer Steps

BODY MEASUREMENTS

Chest 38½   Hips 43

Waist 31¼   Thighs 25¼

Abdomen 38

SUCCESS LEARNING TOOLS

Read pages #

Affirmation

I create my own Joy!
I love exercise!

Other

Plan to Overcome Today's Obstacles:

Take protein bar to eat during afternoon meeting.
Avoid the sweet roll tray.
Drink 30 oz. water mid-day.

Notes:

Call Debbie to ask about Friday's menu.
Request grilled chicken, raw veggies, fruit and lettuce.
Read motivator card before sleep!
Stay focused – it's working!

leanforlife.com

CHOOSE ONE DAY EACH WEEK AS YOUR "PROTEIN DAY."

DAP FOR PROTEIN DAYS

Lean for Life!®

DAILY ACTION PLAN
Protein Day

Week _____ Day _____ Date _____

Time		Serving Size	Carbs (grams)
	Breakfast		
	Protein		
	Beverage		
	Snack		
	Lunch		
	Protein		
	Beverage		
	Snack		
	Dinner		
	Protein		
	Beverage		
	Snack		
		TOTAL	

Keto Reading _____

Weight _____

Vitamin   AM   PM

Water _____

Activities/Duration:
_____
_____

Pedometer Steps _____

BODY MEASUREMENTS

Chest   Hips

Waist   Thighs

Abdomen

SUCCESS LEARNING TOOLS

Read pages # _____

Affirmation _____
_____
_____
_____
_____

Other _____

Plan to Overcome Today's Obstacles:
_____
_____
_____
_____

Notes:
_____
_____
_____
_____
_____
_____
_____

leanforlife.com

DAP FOR MENU DAYS

Lean for Life!®

DAILY ACTION PLAN
Menu Day

Week _____ Day _____ Date _____

Time	Serving Size	Carbs (grams)
Breakfast		
Protein		
Fruit or Grain		
Beverage		
Snack		
Lunch		
Protein		
Vegetable		
Lettuce		
Fruit		
Beverage		
Miscellaneous		
Snack		
Dinner		
Protein		
Vegetable		
Lettuce		
Fruit		
Beverage		
Miscellaneous		
Snack		
	TOTAL	

Keto Reading _____
Weight _____
Vitamin   AM   PM
Water _____

Activities/Duration:

Pedometer Steps _____

BODY MEASUREMENTS

Chest _____   Hips _____
Waist _____   Thighs _____
Abdomen _____

SUCCESS LEARNING TOOLS

Read pages # _____

Affirmation _____

Other _____
Plan to Overcome Today's Obstacles:

Notes:

leanforlife.com

DAP FOR METABOLIC ADJUSTMENT LEVEL 1

Lean for Life!®

METABOLIC ADJUSTMENT
Level 1

Week _____ Day _____ Date _____

Time		Serving Size	Carbs (grams)	Calorie Count
	Breakfast			
	Protein	2			
	Fruit or Grain	1½			
	Beverage	1			
	Snack			
	Lunch			
	Protein	1½			
	Vegetable	1			
	Lettuce	Unl.			
	Fruit	1			
	Beverage	1			
	Miscellaneous	2			
	Snack			
	Dinner			
	Protein	1½			
	Vegetable	1			
	Lettuce	Unl.			
	Fruit	1			
	Beverage	1			
	Miscellaneous	2			
	Snack			
		TOTAL			

Keto Reading   N/A

Weight

Vitamin   AM   PM

Water

Activities/Duration:

Pedometer Steps

BODY MEASUREMENTS

Chest   Hips

Waist   Thighs

Abdomen

SUCCESS LEARNING TOOLS

Read pages #

Affirmation

Other

Plan to Overcome Today's Obstacles:

Notes:

leanforlife.com

DAP FOR METABOLIC ADJUSTMENT LEVEL 2

Lean for Life!®

METABOLIC ADJUSTMENT
Level 2

Week _____ Day _____ Date _____

Time		Serving Size	Carbs (grams)	Calorie Count
	Breakfast			
	Protein	2		
	Fruit or Grain	1½		
	Beverage	1		
	Snack			
	Lunch			
	Protein	2		
	Vegetable	1		
	Lettuce	Unl.		
	Fruit	1		
	Beverage	1		
	Miscellaneous	2		
	Snack			
	Dinner			
	Protein	2		
	Vegetable	1		
	Lettuce	Unl.		
	Fruit	1		
	Beverage	1		
	Miscellaneous	2		
	Snack			
		TOTAL		

Keto Reading   N/A

Weight

Vitamin   AM   PM

Water

Activities/Duration:

\# Pedometer Steps

BODY MEASUREMENTS

Chest   Hips

Waist   Thighs

Abdomen

SUCCESS LEARNING TOOLS

Read pages #

Affirmation

Other

Plan to Overcome Today's Obstacles:

Notes:

leanforlife.com

DAP FOR METABOLIC ADJUSTMENT LEVEL 3

Lean for Life!®

METABOLIC ADJUSTMENT
Level 3

Week _____ Day _____ Date _____

Time		Serving Size	Carbs (grams)	Calorie Count
_____	**Breakfast**			
	Protein	2		
	Fruit or Grain	1½		
	Beverage	1		
_____	**Snack**			
_____	**Lunch**			
	Protein	2		
	Vegetable	1		
	Lettuce	Unl.		
	Fruit	1		
	Grain	1		
	Beverage	1		
	Miscellaneous	2		
_____	**Snack**			
_____	**Dinner**			
	Protein	2		
	Vegetable	1		
	Lettuce	Unl.		
	Fruit	1		
	Grain	1		
	Beverage	1		
	Miscellaneous	2		
_____	**Snack**			
		TOTAL		

Keto Reading   N/A _____
Weight _____
Vitamin   AM   PM _____
Water _____
Activities/Duration: _____
_____
_____

Pedometer Steps _____
BODY MEASUREMENTS
Chest _____ Hips _____
Waist _____ Thighs _____
Abdomen _____
SUCCESS LEARNING TOOLS
Read pages # _____
_____
Affirmation _____
_____
_____
_____
_____
_____
_____
Other _____
Plan to Overcome Today's Obstacles: __
_____
_____
_____
_____
_____
Notes: _____
_____
_____
_____
_____
_____
_____

leanforlife.com

DAP FOR METABOLIC EQUILIBRIUM

Lean for Life!®

DAILY ACTION PLAN
Metabolic Equilibrium

Week _____ Date _____
Day _____ Weight _____

		Protein (grams)	Fat (grams)	Carbs (grams)	Calorie Count
Breakfast	Time:				
Protein					
Fruit					
Grain					
Beverage					
Snack	Time:				
Lunch	Time:				
Protein					
Vegetable					
Lettuce					
Grain					
Fruit					
Beverage					
Miscellaneous					
Snack	Time:				
Dinner	Time:				
Protein					
Vegetable					
Lettuce					
Grain					
Fruit					
Beverage					
Miscellaneous					
Snack	Time:				
TOTAL					

Today I was able to *Eat Better* by...

_____
_____
_____

Today I was able to *Move More* by...

_____
_____
_____

Today I was able to *Stress Less* by...

_____
_____
_____

Today I feel really great about...

_____
_____
_____

Tomorrow I will focus on...

_____
_____
_____

leanforlife.com

DAP FOR AMP

DAY

BREAKFAST

2 Liquid proteins

Food choice:

LUNCH

2 Liquid proteins

Food choice:

SNACK

1 High PER protein bar

Food choice:

DINNER

1 Protein

1 Vegetable

1 Fruit

Food choice:

SNACK

1 Liquid protein

Food choice:

WEIGHT:

KETO READING:

FLUIDS:

EXERCISE:

FAQS ABOUT AMP

Want more information about the AMP plateau-busting plan?
Check out these FAQs.

Why were these foods selected?

These foods are low in calories, low in carbohydrates and low glycemic.

What is the daily carbohydrate count?

It ranges from 50 to 65.

Why is dinner my only meal?

Pre-measured protein foods with minimal preparation time, along with a balanced meal for dinner, was designed for convenience.

If this works for me, can I stay on the AMP plan longer?

No, the AMP is a tool used once during the Rapid Weight Loss phase for a few days. This food plan does not provide adequate nutrition for a longer term.

Can Miscellaneous foods be used on the AMP?

Miscellaneous foods, such as fat-free, non-dairy powdered coffee creamer with coffee or two radishes with the dinner lettuce, may be used.

Can the fiber drinks and fiber gelatin be used while on the AMP?

Yes.

Do I need to consume both liquid proteins at breakfast and at lunch?

Yes, the two liquid proteins must be consumed together at breakfast and at lunch.

WHAT ARE LEAN FOR LIFE HIGH PER PROTEIN PRODUCTS?

In addition to the many food choices included under "Proteins" in the "Lean Foods" lists, you may use any of the Lean for Life high protein-efficiency ratio (PER) protein nutritional products during your program. These high PER protein, low-carbohydrate, low-calorie products have been specifically designed for use in all phases of the program and may be used as the protein portion of meals, as a snack and on Protein Days.

While it's entirely realistic for you to succeed on the program without using any of the Lean for Life products mentioned in this book, using them can enhance your experience by providing more of what the program is all about: choices. The Lean for Life product line offers dozens of options, ranging from only 1 to 16 grams of "usable" carbs per serving.

The Lean for Life product line is ever changing and offers something for every appetite, including the following.

- **Protein bars:** These delicious protein bars are available in a variety of flavors, including Peanut Butter Crunch, Lemon Meringue, Dark Chocolate S'mores, Double Chocolate, Chocolate Mint, Oatmeal Cinnamon Raisin, Dark Chocolate Coated Coconut and Crisp 'N Crunch Double Berry Breakfast.

- **Shakes, smoothies and puddings:** Choose from a selection of shakes in such flavors as Creamy Vanilla, Creamy Chocolate and Mocha; smoothies come in flavors such as Berry Creme, Mango and Café Latte; and puddings come in flavors such as Dulce de Leche, Lemon Chiffon and Custard Creme with Toffee Bits.

- **Fruit-flavored cold drinks:** Flavors like Peach Mango, Wildberry Passion and Strawberry Kiwi are nutritious and delicious.

- **Hot drinks:** Creamy Hot Cocoa, Cappuccino and Raspberry Hot Cocoa are among our best-selling hot drinks.

- **Hot soups:** Choose from such favorites as Chicken Noodle, Cream of Chicken with Vegetables, Cream of Tomato and Cream of Mushroom.

- **Hot dishes:** Selections include Macaroni & Cheese, Vegetable Chili, Vegetable Spaghetti, Nacho Cheese Pasta, Vegetarian Sloppy Joe, and Oatmeal with Apples and Cinnamon.

- **Crunchy snacks:** Barbeque Crunch O's, Crunchy BBQ Soy Puffs, Cheddar Cheese Double Bites, Crunchy Chili, Lime Soy Puffs, Chocolate Chip Cookies and Dark Chocolate Tea Biscuits.

- **Frozen items:** KOT Crèpes and KOT Pizza.

You may notice that many of the Lean for Life nutritional products include "total" carbs and "usable" carbs on the nutrition labels. What's the difference, and which do you track? Many of the Lean for Life nutritional products contain ingredients that are classified as carbohydrates but that cannot be fully absorbed and "used" by the body. Even though these ingredients are not fully used by the body, they must be included in the "total carbs" number listed on the product's nutrition label. For example, the product label may show the "total carbs" number as 14 grams while the number of carbs your body actually "uses" may be only 8 grams. When the "usable" carbs number is provided, this is the number you need to track. On all other products and foods, you'll keep track of the "total carbs" number.

View the latest Lean for Life high PER protein products.

APPENDIX C

GLYCEMIC INDEX CHART

The Glycemic Index (GI) ranks foods on a scale of 1 to 100 based on how they affect blood sugar and insulin levels. The higher the ranking number, the greater the increase in blood sugar and insulin levels. The lower the number, the lower the impact on blood sugar and insulin. In this chart, rankings have been rounded up or down to multiples of 5.

HIGH GI (NOT FOR RAPID WEIGHT LOSS!)

100	Glucose
95	Baked potato, French fries, rice cakes
90	Honey, mashed potatoes, pasta (overcooked)
85	Popcorn, pretzels, white bread
80	Broad beans, crackers, gingerbread, oatmeal (instant), tapioca
75	Baguette, pumpkin, white bread
70	Boiled potatoes, corn, croissants, white rice

MODERATE GI

65	Cantaloupe, Kashi Puffs, melon, Nutri-Grain, pineapple, raisins
60	Bananas, grapes, papaya
55	All-Bran, quinoa

GLYCEMIC INDEX CHART

LOW GI

50	Brown rice, kiwis, oatmeal (steel cut or slow cooking), whole-grain bread
45	Grapes
40	Oranges, peaches, pears, raspberries, strawberries
35	Apples, carrots (raw), yogurt (nonfat, plain)
30	Skim milk
25	Grapefruit
20	Cherries
15	Apricots
10	Dark leafy greens, green vegetables, lettuce, mushrooms, onions, peppers, tomatoes

APPENDIX D

BODY MASS INDEX (BMI) CHART

Find your height in the left-hand column, then read across that row to find your weight. Your BMI is at the top of that column.

BMI	Under-weight	Healthy Weight					Overweight					Obese		Morbidly Obese
	19	20	21	22	23	24	25	26	27	28	29	30	35	40
4'10"	91	96	100	105	110	115	119	124	129	134	138	143	167	191
4'11"	94	99	104	109	114	119	124	128	133	138	143	148	173	198
5'0"	97	102	107	112	118	123	128	133	138	143	148	153	179	204
5'1"	100	106	111	116	122	127	132	137	143	148	153	158	185	211
5'2"	104	109	115	120	126	131	136	142	147	153	158	164	191	218
5'3"	107	113	118	124	130	135	141	146	152	158	163	169	197	225
5'4"	110	116	122	128	134	140	145	151	157	163	169	174	204	232
5'5"	114	120	126	132	138	144	150	156	162	168	174	180	210	240
5'6"	118	124	130	136	142	148	155	161	167	173	179	186	216	247
5'7"	121	127	134	140	146	153	159	166	172	178	185	191	223	255
5'8"	125	131	138	144	151	158	164	171	177	184	190	197	230	262
5'9"	128	135	142	149	155	162	169	176	182	189	196	203	236	270
5'10"	132	139	146	153	160	167	174	181	188	195	202	207	243	278
5'11"	136	143	150	157	165	172	179	186	193	200	208	215	250	286
6'0"	140	147	154	162	169	177	184	191	199	206	213	221	258	294
6'1"	144	151	159	166	174	182	189	197	204	212	219	227	265	302
6'2"	148	155	163	171	179	186	194	202	210	218	225	233	272	311
6'3"	152	160	168	176	184	192	200	208	216	224	232	240	279	319
6'4"	156	164	172	180	189	197	205	213	221	230	238	246	287	328

APPENDIX E

STARTING MEASUREMENTS

IDEAL LEAN WEIGHT GOAL:	
CURRENT WEIGHT:	(to nearest 1/2 pound)

BODY MEASUREMENTS
(to nearest ¼ inch)

WAIST:	
CHEST:	
LOWER ABDOMEN:	
HIPS:	
UPPER THIGH AREA:	
BMI:	
WAIST-TO-HEIGHT RATIO:	

APPENDIX F

WEEKLY PROGRESS REPORT: HOW ARE YOU DOING?

WEIGHT:
(to nearest 1/2 pound)

BODY MEASUREMENTS
(to nearest $\frac{1}{4}$ inch)

WAIST:

CHEST:

LOWER ABDOMEN:

HIPS:

UPPER THIGH AREA:

BMI:

WAIST-TO-HEIGHT RATIO:

On a scale of 1-10 with 1 being poor and 10 being fantastic, rate your average level for:

EATING BETTER THIS WEEK:

MOVING MORE THIS WEEK:

STRESSING LESS THIS WEEK:

WEEKLY PROGRESS REPORT:
HOW ARE YOU DOING?

Rate your average inner sabotage agent alert level: (check one)

ABOUT THE SAME:

GETTING BETTER:

GETTING WORSE:

Rate your ability to practice thought control: (check one)

ABOUT THE SAME:

GETTING BETTER:

GETTING WORSE:

Rate your cravings in terms of intensity and frequency: (check one)

ABOUT THE SAME:

FEWER CRAVINGS AND/OR LESS INTENSE:

MORE CRAVINGS AND/OR MORE INTENSE:

APPENDIX G

WOMEN—"HOW MUCH CAN I EAT?"

ACTIVE (6,000 steps or more per day)
12–14 calories per pound of body weight

Weight	Calories per day	Carbohydrates–45% 1 gram = 4 cal Calories / Grams	Protein–25% 1 gram = 4 cal Calories / Grams	Fat–30% or less 1 gram = 9 cal Calories / Grams
100 lb.	1,200-1,400	540-630 / 135-158	300-350 / 75-88	360-420 / 40-47
120 lb.	1,440-1,680	648-756 / 162-189	360-420 / 90-105	432-504 / 48-56
140 lb.	1,680-1,960	756-882 / 189-221	420-490 / 105-123	504-588 / 56-65
160 lb.	1,920-2,240	864-1,008 / 216-252	480-560 / 120-140	576-672 / 64-75

INACTIVE (Fewer than 6,000 steps per day)
10–12 calories per pound of body weight

Weight	Calories per day	Carbohydrates–45% 1 gram = 4 cal Calories / Grams	Protein–25% 1 gram = 4 cal Calories / Grams	Fat–30% or less 1 gram = 9 cal Calories / Grams
100 lb.	1,000-1,200	450-540 / 113-135	250-300 / 63-75	300-360 / 33-40
120 lb.	1,200-1,440	540-648 / 135-162	300-360 / 75-90	360-432 / 40-48
140 lb.	1,400-1,680	630-756 / 158-189	350-420 / 88-105	420-504 / 47-56
160 lb.	1,600-1,920	720-864 / 180-216	400-480 / 100-120	480-576 / 53-64

MEN—"HOW MUCH CAN I EAT?"

ACTIVE (6,000 steps or more per day)
14-16 calories per pound of body weight

Weight	Calories per day	Carbohydrates–45% 1 gram = 4 cal Calories / Grams	Protein–25% 1 gram = 4 cal Calories / Grams	Fat–30% or less 1 gram = 9 cal Calories / Grams
150 lb.	2,100-2,400	945-1,080 / 236-270	525-600 / 131-150	630-720 / 70-80
170 lb.	2,380-2,720	1,071-1,224 / 268-306	595-680 / 149-170	714-816 / 79-91
190 lb.	2,660-3,040	1,197-1,368 / 299-342	665-760 / 166-190	798-912 / 89-101
210 lb.	2,940-3,360	1,323-1,512 / 331-378	735-840 / 184-210	882-1,008 / 98-112

INACTIVE (Fewer than 6,000 steps per day)
12-14 calories per pound of body weight

150 lb.	1,800-2,100	810-945 / 203-236	450-525 / 113-131	540-630 / 60-70
170 lb.	2,040-2,380	918-1,071 / 230-268	510-595 / 128-149	612-714 / 68-79
190 lb.	2,280-2,660	1,026-1,197 / 257-299	570-665 / 143-166	684-798 / 76-89
210 lb.	2,520-2,940	1,134-1,323 / 284-331	630-735 / 158-184	756-882 / 84-98

REFERENCES

INTRODUCTION

Buckland, Danny. 2012. "On a Hiding to No-Thin: Half of Dieters Give Up After a Month." *Mirror*, November 5.

CHAPTER 1

Ainslie, Deborah A., Joseph Proietto, Barbara C. Fam, and Anne W. Thorburn. 2000. "Short-Term, High-Fat Diets Lower Circulating Leptin Concentrations in Rats." *American Journal of Clinical Nutrition* 71(2):438–42. http://ajcn.nutrition.org/content/71/2/438.full.

Allouche, Réginald, and Florence Massiéra. *Mincir A Satiété: La Nouvelle Méthode Pour Reprogrammer Votre Appétit* (Paris: Flammarion, 2009), 53–78.

Chaudhari, Nirupa, and Stephen D. Roper. 2010. "The Cell Biology of Taste." *The Journal of Cell Biology* 190(3):285–96. doi:10.1083/jcb.201003144.

Eberle, Ute. 2012. "Le Fabuleux Destin d'une Bouchée de Pizza." Translated by Emmanuel Basset. *GEO Savoir*, September/October, 66–83.

Goldstone, Tony. 2010. "Stomach Hormone Ghrelin Increases Desire for High-Calorie Foods." Paper presented at the Annual Meeting of the Endocrine Society, San Diego, CA, June 19–22.

Kirchner, Henriette, Jesus A. Gutierrez, Patricia J. Solenberg, Paul T. Pfluger, Traci A. Czyzyk, Jill A. Willency, Annette Shürmann, et al. 2009. "GOAT Links Dietary Lipids with the Endocrine Control of Energy Balance." *Nature Medicine* 15:741–45. doi:10.1038/nm.1997.

Kokkinos, Alexander, Carel W. le Roux, Kleopatra Alexiadou, Nicholas Tentolouris, Royce P. Vincent, Despoina Kyriaki, Despoina Perrea, et al. 2010. "Eating Slowly Increases the Postprandial Response of the Anorexigenic Gut Hormones, Peptide YY and Glucagon-Like Peptide-1." *The Journal of Clinical Endocrinology & Metabolism* 95(1):333–37. doi:10.1210/jc.2009-1018.

Koutatsu, Maruyama, Shinichi Sato, Tetsuya Ohira, Kenji Maeda, Hiroyuki Noda, Yoshimi Kubota, Setsuko Nishimura, et al. 2008. "The Joint Impact on Being Overweight of Self Reported Behaviours of Eating Quickly and Eating Until Full: Cross Sectional Survey." *British Medical Journal* 337:a2002. http://dx.doi.org/10.1136/bmj.a2002.

Li, Jie, Na Zhang, Lizhen Hu, Ze Li, Rui Li, Cong Li, and Shuran Wang. 2011. "Improvement in Chewing Activity Reduces Energy Intake in One Meal and Modulates Plasma Gut Hormone Concentrations in Obese and Lean Young Chinese Men." *American Journal of Clinical Nutrition* 94(3):709–16. doi:10.3945/ajcn.111.015164.

Oswal, Ashwini, and Giles Yeo. 2010. "Leptin and the Control of Body Weight: A Review of Its Diverse Central Targets, Signaling Mechanisms, and Role in the Pathogenesis of Obesity." *Obesity* 18:221–29. doi:10.1038/oby.2009.228.

Rodríguez, Amaia, Javier Gómez-Ambrosi, Victoria Catalán, Maria J. Gil, Sara Becerril, Neria Sáinz, Camilo Sliva, et al. 2009. "Acylated and Desacyl Ghrelin Stimulate Lipid Accumulation in Human Visceral Adipocytes Lipogenic Effect of Ghrelin in Humans." *International Journal of Obesity* 33:541–52. doi:10.1038/ijo.2009.40.

Zimmerman, Kim Ann. 2012. "Circulatory System: Facts, Functions & Diseases." *LiveScience*. Last modified August 17. www.livescience.com/22486-circulatory-system.html.

CHAPTER 2

Bistrian, Bruce R. 1978. "Clinical Use of a Protein-Sparing Modified Fast." *Journal of the American Medical Association* 240(21):2299–2302. http://jama.jamanetwork.com/article.aspx?articleid=362377.

Blackburn, George L., and Isaac Greenberg. 1978. "Multidisciplinary Approach to Adult Obesity Therapy." *International Journal of Obesity* 2(2):133–42. www.ncbi.nlm.nih.gov/pubmed/711360.

Hoffer, Leonard J., Bruce R. Bistrian, Vernon R. Young, George L. Blackburn, and Dwight E. Matthews. 1984. "Metabolic Effects of Very Low Calorie Weight Restriction Diets." *The Journal of Clinical Investigation* 73(3):750–58. doi:10.1172/JCI111268.

Hooper, Lee, Asmaa Abdelhamid, Helen J. Moore, Wayne Douthwaite, C. Muray Skeaff, and Carolyn D. Summerbell. 2012. "Effect of Reducing Total Fat Intake on

Body Weight: Systematic Review and Meta-Analysis of Randomised Controlled Trials and Cohort Studies." *British Medical Journal* 345:e7666. doi:10.1136/bmj.e7666.

Kennedy, Adam R., Pavlos Pissios, Hasan Otu, Bingzhong Xue, Kenji Asakura, Noboru Furukawa, Frank E. Marino, et al. 2007. "A High-Fat, Ketogenic Diet Induces a Unique Metabolic State in Mice." *American Journal of Physiology—Endocrinology and Metabolism* 292:E1724–39. doi:10.1152/ajpendo.00717.2006.

Palgi, Aviva, Leighton Read, Isaac Greenberg, Martha A. Hoefer, Bruce R. Bistrian, and George L. Blackburn. 1985. "Multidisciplinary Treatment of Obesity with a Protein-Sparing Modified Fast: Results in 668 Outpatients." *American Journal of Public Health* 75(10): 1190–94. www.ncbi.nlm.nih.gov/pmc/articles/PMC1646394/.

Phinney, Stephen D., Bruce R. Bistrian, Robert R. Wolfe, and George L. Blackburn. 1983. "The Human Metabolic Response to Chronic Ketosis Without Calorie Restriction: Physical and Biochemical Adaptation." *Metabolism* 32(8):757–68. http://dx.doi.org/10.1016/0026-0495(83)90105-1.

Shimazu, Tadahiro, Matthew D. Hirschey, John Newman, Wenjuan He, Kotaro Shirakawa, Natacha Le Moan, Carrie A. Grueter, et al. 2012. "Suppression of Oxidative Stress by β-Hydroxybutyrate, an Endogenous Histone Deacetylase Inhibitor." *Science* 339(6116): 211–14. doi:10.1126/science.1227166.

CHAPTER 3

Ansell, Emily B., Kenneth Rando, Keri Tuit, Joseph Guarnaccia, and Rajita Sinha. 2012. "Cumulative Adversity and Smaller Gray Matter Volume in Medial Prefrontal, Anterior Cingulate, and Insula Regions." *Biological Psychiatry* 72(1):57–64. doi: 10.1016/j.biopsych.2011.11.022.

Brooks, Samantha J., Christian Benedict, Jonathan Burgos, Matthew J. Kempton, Richard Nordenskjöld, Lena Kilander, Ruta Nylander, et al. 2013. "Late-Life Obesity Is Associated with Smaller Global and Regional Gray Matter Volumes: A Voxel-Based Morphometric Study." *International Journal of Obesity* 37(2):230–36. doi:10.1038/ijo.2012.13.

Brown, Christopher A., and Anthony K. P. Jones. 2010. "Meditation Experience Predicts Less Negative Appraisal of Pain: Electrophysiological Evidence for the Involvement of Anticipatory Neural Responses." *Pain* 150(3):428–38. doi:10.1016/j.pain.2010.04.017.

Watkins, Lana L., Gary G. Koch, Andrew Sherwood, James A. Blumenthal, Jonathan R. T. Davidson, Christopher O'Connor, and Michael H. Sketch. 2013. "Association of Anxiety and Depression with All-Cause Mortality in Individuals with Coronary Heart Disease." *Journal of the American Heart Association* 2(2):e000068. doi:10.1161/JAHA.112.000068.

CHAPTER 4

DAY 1

Duraffourd, Celine, Filipe De Vadder, Daisy Goncalves, Fabien Delaere, Armelle Penhoat, Bluenn Brusset, Fabienne Rajas, et al. 2012. "Mu-Opioid Receptors and Dietary Protein Stimulate a Gut-Brain Neural Circuitry Limiting Food Intake." *Cell* 150(2):377–88. doi:10.1016/j.cell.2012.05.039.

Rizkalla, Salwa W., Edi Prifti, Aurélie Cotillard, Véronique Pelloux, Christine Rouault, Réginald Allouche, Muriel Laromiguière, et al. 2012. "Differential Effects of Macronutrient Content in 2 Energy-Restricted Diets on Cardiovascular Risk Factors and Adipose Tissue Cell Size in Moderately Obese Individuals: A Randomized Controlled Trial." *American Journal of Clinical Nutrition* 95(1):49–63. doi: 10.3945/ajcn.111.017277.

DAY 2

Rubin, Theodore Isaac. *Forever Thin* (New York: B. Geis Associates, 1970), 21.

DAY 3

Cobb-Clark, Deborah A., Sonja C. Kassenboehmer, and Stefanie Shurer. 2012. "Healthy Habits: The Connection Between Diet, Exercise, and Locus of Control." Working Paper No. 15/12, ISSN 1328-4991, *Melbourne Institute Working Paper Series*, Melbourne, Australia. www.melbourneinstitute.com/downloads/working_paper_series/wp2012n15.pdf.

Forman, Evan M., Meghan Butryn, Adrienne S. Juarascio, Lauren E. Bradley, Mackenzie Kelly, Ami P. Belmont, Michael R. Lowe, et al. 2012. "A Randomized Controlled Trial Comparing Gold Standard and Acceptance-based Behavioral Treatment for Obesity: Outcomes from the Mind Your Health Program." Poster presented at the 30th Annual Obesity Society Scientific Meeting, San Antonio, TX, September 20–24.

Li, Jie, Na Zhang, Lizhen Hu, Ze Li, Rui Li, Cong Li, and Shuran Wang. 2011. "Improvement in Chewing Activity Reduces Energy Intake in One Meal and Modulates Plasma Gut Hormone Concentrations in Obese and Lean Young Chinese Men." *American Journal of Clinical Nutrition* 94(3):709–16. doi:10.3945/ajcn.111.015164.

Mithieux, Gilles, Pierre Misery, Christophe Magnan, Bruno Pillot, Amandine Gautier-Stein, Christine Bernard, Fabienne Rajas, and Carine Zitoun. 2005. "Portal Sensing of Intestinal Gluconeogenesis is a Mechanistic Link in the Diminution of Food Intake Induced by Diet Protein." *Cell Metabolism* 2(5):321–29. doi:10.1016/j.cmet.2005.09.010.

Neal, David T., Wendy Wood, and Jeffrey M. Quinn. 2006. "Habits—A Repeat Performance." *Current Directions in Psychological Science* 15(4):198–202. doi: 10.1111/j.1467-8721.2006.00435.x.

Xu, Xiaomeng, Tricia M. Leahey, and Rena R. Wing. 2012. "The Power of Tenacity: Behavioral Perseverance is Associated With Successful Weight Loss and Increases in Physical Activity." Paper presented at the 30th Annual Obesity Society Scientific Meeting, San Antonio, Texas, September 20–24.

DAY 5

Yu, Xinjun, Masaki Fumoto, Yasushi Nakatani, Tamami Sekiyama, Hiromi Kikuchi, Yoshinari Seki, Ikuko Sato-Suzuki, et al. 2011. "Activation of the Anterior Prefrontal Cortex and Serotonergic System is Associated with Improvements in Mood and EEG Changes Induced by Zen Meditation Practice in Novices." *International Journal of Psychophysiology* 80(2):103–11. doi: 10.1016/j.ijpsycho.2011.02.004.

DAY 7

Andrade, Flavia Cristina Drumond, Marcela Raffaelli, Margarita Teran-Garcia, Jilber A. Jerman, Celia Aradillas Garcia, and Up Amigos 2009 Study Group. 2012. "Weight Status Misperception Among Mexican Young Adults." *Body Image* 9(1):184–88. doi: 10.1016/j.bodyim.2011.10.006.

Rizkalla, Salwa W., Edi Prifti, Aurélie Cotillard, Véronique Pelloux, Christine Rouault, Réginald Allouche, Muriel Laromiguière, LingChun Kong, Froogh Darakhshan, Florence Massiera, and Karine Clement. 2012. "Differential Effects of Macronutrient Content in 2 Energy-Restricted Diets on Cardiovascular Risk Factors and Adipose

Tissue Cell Size in Moderately Obese Individuals: A Randomized Controlled Trial." *American Journal of Clinical Nutrition* 95(1):49–63. doi: 10.3945/ajcn.111.017277.

CHAPTER 5

DAY 8

Allouche, Réginald, and Florence Massiéra. *Mincir A Satiété: La Nouvelle Méthode Pour Reprogrammer Votre Appétit* (Paris: Flammarion, 2009), 53–78.

Borzoei, S., M. Neovius, B. Barkeline, A. Teixera-Pinto, and S. Rossner. 2006. "A Comparison of Effects of Fish and Beef Protein on Satiety in Normal Weight Men." *European Journal of Clinical Nutrition* 60(7):897–902. www.ncbi.nlm.nih.gov/pubmed/16482079.

Briggs, Dana I., Pablo J. Enriori, Moyra B. Lemus, Michael A. Cowley, and Zane B. Andrews. 2010. "Diet-Induced Obesity Causes Ghrelin Resistance in Arcuate NPY/Agrp Neurons." *Endocrinology* 151(10):4745–55. doi:10.1210/en.2010-0556.

Diz-Chaves, Yolanda. 2011. "Ghrelin, Appetite Regulation, and Food Reward: Interaction with Chronic Stress." *International Journal of Peptides* (2011): Article ID 898450. doi:10.1155/2011/898450.

Faipoux, Rodolphe, Daniel Tomé, Ahmed Bensaid, Céline Morens, Eric Oriol, Laurent Michel Bonnano, and Gilles Fromentin. 2006. "Yeast Proteins Enhance Satiety in Rats." *The Journal of Nutrition* 136(9):2350–56. http://jn.nutrition.org/content/136/9/2350.long.

Faipoux, Rodolphe, Daniel Tomé, Sylvette Gougis, Nicolas Darcel, and Gilles Fromentin. 2008. "Proteins Activate Satiety-Related Neuronal Pathways in the Brainstem and Hypothalamus of Rats." *The Journal of Nutrition* 138(6):1172–78. http://jn.nutrition.org/content/138/6/1172.long.

Gannon, Mary C., and Frank Q. Nuttall. 2011. "Effect of a High-Protein Diet on Ghrelin, Growth Hormone, and Insulin-Like Growth Factor-I and Binding Proteins 1 and 3 in Subjects With Type 2 Diabetes Mellitus." *Metabolism* 60(9):1300–11. doi:10.1016/j.metabol.2011.01.016.

Goldstone, Tony. 2010. "Stomach Hormone Ghrelin Increases Desire for High-Calorie Foods." Paper presented at the 92nd Annual Meeting of the Endocrine Society, San Diego, CA, June 19–22.

Luhovyy, Bohdan L., Tina Akhavan, and G. Harvey Anderson. 2007. "Whey Proteins in the Regulation of Food Intake and Satiety." *Journal of the American College of Nutrition* 26(6):704S–12S. www.jacn.org/content/26/6/704S.long.

Pichon, Lisa, Mylène Potier, Daniel Tomé, Takashi Mikogami, Benoit Laplaize, Christine Martin-Rouas, and Gilles Fromentin. 2008. "High-Protein Diets Containing Different Milk Protein Fractions Differently Influence Energy Intake and Adiposity in the Rat." *British Journal of Nutrition* 99(4):739–48. ncbi.nlm.nih.gov/pubmed/18005480.

Rodríguez, Amaia, Javier Gómez-Ambrosi, Victoria Catalán, Maria J. Gil, Sara Becerril, Neria Sáinz, Camilo Sliva, et al. 2009. "Acylated and Desacyl Ghrelin Stimulate Lipid Accumulation in Human Visceral Adipocytes Lipogenic Effect of Ghrelin in Humans." *International Journal of Obesity* 33:541–52. doi:10.1038/ijo.2009.40.

Tillisch, Kirsten, Jennifer Labus, Lisa Kilpatrick, Zhiguo Jiang, Jean Stains, Bahar Ebrat, Denis Guyonnet, et al. 2013. "Consumption of Fermented Milk Product with Probiotic Modulates Brain Activity." *Gastroenterology* 144 (7): 1394–401. doi:10.1053/j.gastro.2013.02.043.

Tomé, Daniel, Jessica Schwarz, Nicolas Darcel, and Gilles Fromentin. 2009. "Protein, Amino Acids, Vagus Nerve Signaling, and the Brain." *American Journal of Clinical Nutrition* 90 (Suppl): 838S–843S. doi:10.3945/ajcn.2009.27462W.

Westerterp-Plantenga, Margriet S., Sofie G. Lemmens, and Klaas R. Westerterp. 2012. "Dietary Protein—Its Role in Satiety, Energetics, Weight Loss and Health." *British Journal of Nutrition* 108 (Suppl 2): S105–S112. doi:10.1017/S0007114512002589.

DAY 9

Quinn, Timothy J., and Benjamin A. Coons. 2011. "The Talk Test and Its Relationship with the Ventilatory and Lactate Thresholds." *Journal of Sports* 29(11):1175–82. doi: 10.1080/02640414.2011.585165.

Wen, Chi Pang, Jackson Pui Man Wai, Min Kuang Tsai, Yi Chen Yang, Ting Yuan David Cheng, Meng-Chih Lee, Hui Ting Chan, et al. 2011. "Minimum Amount of Physical Activity for Reduced Mortality and Extended Life Expectancy: A Prospective Cohort Study." *The Lancet* 378 (9798): 1244–53. doi:10.1016/S0140-6736(11)60749-6.

Williams, Paul T., and Paul D. Thompson. 2013. "Walking Versus Running for Hypertension, Cholesterol, and Diabetes Mellitus Risk Reduction." *Arteriosclerosis, Thrombosis and Vascular Biology* 33:1085–91. doi: 10.1161/ATVBAHA.112.300878.

DAY 10

American Psychological Association. 2012. The Stress in America™ survey. (Washington, D.C.: American Psychological Association).

Bailey, Michael T., Scot E. Dowd, Jeffrey D. Galley, Amy R. Hufnagle, Rebecca G. Allen, and Mark Lyte. 2011. "Exposure to a Social Stressor Alters the Structure of the Intestinal Microbiota: Implications for Stressor-Induced Immunomodulation." *Brain, Behavior, and Immunity* 25(3):397–407. doi:10.1016/j.bbi.2010.10.023.

Kiecolt-Glaser, Janice K., Martha A. Belury, Rebecca Andridge, William B. Malarkey, and Ronald Glaser. 2011. "Omega-3 Supplementation Lowers Inflammation and Anxiety in Medical Students: A Randomized Controlled Trial." *Brain, Behavior, and Immunity* 25(8):1725–34. doi: 10.1016/j.bbi.2011.07.229.

Rapaport, Mark Hyman, Pamela Schettler, and Catherine Bresee. 2010. "A Preliminary Study of the Effects of a Single Session of Swedish Massage on Hypothalamic-Pituitary-Adrenal and Immune Function in Normal Individuals." *The Journal of Alternative and Complementary Medicine* 16(10):1079–88. doi:10.1089/acm.2009.0634.

DAY 11

Allouche, Réginald. *La Révolution Minceur* (Paris: Michel Lafon, 2003), 65–67.

Allouche, Réginald, and Florence Massiéra. *Mincir A Satiété: La Nouvelle Méthode Pour Reprogrammer Votre Appétit* (Paris: Flammarion, 2009), 73–77.

Clement, Karine, and Dominique Langin. 2007. "Regulation of Inflammation-Related Genes in Human Adipose Tissue." *Journal of Internal Medicine* 262:422–30. doi: 10.1111/j.1365-2796.2007.01851.x.

Deng, Tuo, Christopher J. Lyon, Laurie J. Minze, Jianxin Lin, Jia Zou, Joey Z. Liu, Yuelan Ren, et al. 2013. "Class II Major Histocompatibility Complex Plays an Essential Role in Obesity-Induced Adipose Inflammation." *Cell Metabolism* 17(3):411–22. doi: 10.1016/j.cmet.2013.02.009.

Massiera, Florence, Pascal Barbry, Philippe Guesnet, Aurélie Joly, Serge Luquet, Chimène Moreilhon-Brest, Tala Mohsen-Kanson, et al. 2010. "A Western-Like Fat Diet Is Sufficient to Induce a Gradual Enhancement in Fat Mass Over Generations." *Journal of Lipid Research* 51:2352–61. doi:10.1194/jlr.M006866.

Miller, Carla K., Jean L. Kristeller, Amy Headings, Haikady Nagaraja, and W. Fred Miser. 2012. "Comparative Effectiveness of a Mindful Eating Intervention to a

Diabetes Self-Management Intervention among Adults with Type 2 Diabetes: A Pilot Study." *Journal of the Academy of Nutrition and Dietetics* 112 (11): 1835. doi:10.1016/j.jand.2012.07.036.

Müller, Timo D., Sang Jun Lee, Martin Jastroch, Dhiraj Kabra, Kerstin Stemmer, Michaela Aichler, Bill Abplanalp, et al. 2012. "p62 Links β-Adrenergic Input to Mitochondrial Function and Thermogenesis." *Journal of Clinical Investigation* 123(1):469. doi:10.1172/JCI64209.

Rizkalla, Salwa W., Edi Prifti, Aurélie Cotillard, Véronique Pelloux, Christine Rouault, Réginald Allouche, Muriel Laromiguière, et al. 2012. "Differential Effects of Macronutrient Content in 2 Energy-Restricted Diets on Cardiovascular Risk Factors and Adipose Tissue Cell Size in Moderately Obese Individuals: A Randomized Controlled Trial." *The American Journal of Clinical Nutrition* 95(1):49–63. doi:10.3945/ajcn.111.017277.

Robinson, Eric, Paul Aveyard, Amanda Daley, Kate Jolly, Amanda Lewis, Deborah Lycett, and Suzanne Higgs. 2013. "Eating Attentively: A Systematic Review and Meta-analysis of the Effect of Food Intake Memory and Awareness on Eating." *The American Journal of Clinical Nutrition* 97(4):728–42. doi: 10.3945/ajcn.112.045245.

Saltiel, Alan R. 2001. "You Are What You Secrete." *Nature Medicine* 7:887–88. doi:10.1038/90911.

Valet, Philippe. 2009. "Le Tissue Adipeux et Ses Hormones." *Pour La Science*, October. www.pourlascience.fr/ewb_pages/f/fiche-article-le-tissu-adipeux-et-ses-hormones-23441.php.

Wansink, Brian. *Mindless Eating: Why We Eat More Than We Think* (New York: Dell, 2006).

DAY 12

Atkinson, Fiona S., Kaye Foster-Powell, and Jennie C. Brand-Miller. 2008. "International Tables of Glycemic Index and Glycemic Load Values." *Diabetes Care* 31(12):2281–83. doi:10.2337/dc08-1239.

Lin, Ching-I, Wan-Teng Lin, Ming-Jen Fan, Ming-Chang Lin, Chang-Hai Tsai, Fuu-Jen Tsai, Wei-Jen Ting, et al. 2011. "Clinical Characteristics Change and the Heart Rate Variability of Subjects with Metabolic Syndrome in the Weight Loss Program." Proceedings of the 2011 IEEE 11th International Conference on Bioinformatics and Bioengineering, Taichung, Taiwan, October 24–26, 155–61. doi: 10.1109/BIBE.2011.66.

Murad, Khalil, Peter H. Brubaker, David M. Fitzgerald, Timothy M. Morgan, David C. Goff, Elsayed Z. Soliman, Joel D. Eggebeen, et al. 2012. "Exercise Training Improves Heart Rate Variability in Older Patients with Heart Failure: A Randomized, Controlled, Single-Blinded Trial." *Congestive Heart Failure* 18:192–97. doi:10.1111/j.1751-7133.2011.00282.x.

Routledge, Faye S., Tavis S. Campbell, Judith A. McFertidge-Durdle, and Simon L. Bacon. 2010. "Improvements in Heart Rate Variability with Exercise Therapy." *The Canadian Journal of Cardiology* 26(6):303–12. www.ncbi.nlm.nih.gov/pmc/articles/PMC2903986/.

Sjoberg, Nicholas, Grant D. Brinkworth, Thomas P. Wycherley, Manny Noakes, and David A. Saint. 2011. "Moderate Weight Loss Improves Heart Rate Variability in Overweight and Obese Adults with Type 2 Diabetes." *Journal of Applied Physiology* 110(4):1060–64. doi:10.1152/japplphysiol.01329.2010.

DAY 13

Blumenthal, James A., Michael A. Babyak, P. Murali Doraiswamy, Lana Watkins, Benson M. Hoffman, Krista A. Barbour, Steve Herman, et al. 2007. "Exercise and Pharmacotherapy in the Treatment of Major Depressive Disorder." *Psychosomatic Medicine* 69(7):587–96. doi:10.1097/PSY.0b013e318148c19a.

Bravo, Javier A., Paul Forsythe, Marianne V. Chew, Emily Escaravage, Hélène M. Savignac, Timothy G. Dinan, John Bienenstock, and John F. Cryan. 2011. "Ingestion of Lactobacillus Strain Regulates Emotional Behavior and Central GABA Receptor Expression in a Mouse Via the Vagus Nerve." Proceedings of the National Academy of Sciences 108(38):16050–55. doi:10.1073/pnas.1102999108.

Hoffman, Benson M., Michael A. Babyak, W. Edward Craighead, Andrew Sherwood, P. Murali Doraiswamy, Michael J. Coons, and James A. Blumenthal. 2011. "Exercise and Pharmacotherapy in Patients with Major Depression: One-Year Follow-Up of the SMILE Study." *Psychosomatic Medicine* 73(2):127–33. doi:10.1097/PSY.0b013e31820433a5.

Maes, Michael, Marta Kubera, and Jean-Claude Leunis. 2008. "The Gut-Brain Barrier in Major Depression: Intestinal Mucosal Dysfunction with an Increased Translocation of LPS from Gram Negative Enterobacteria (Leaky Gut) Plays a Role in the Inflammatory Pathophysiology of Depression." *Neuroendocrinology Letters* 29(1):117–24. https://level4now.com/image/data/Clinical-Studies/dodrops/Gut-BrainBarrierInMajorDepression%26InflammatoryPathophysiologyOfDepression.pdf.

Mojtabai, Ramin, and Mark Olfson. 2011. "Proportion of Antidepressants Prescribed Without a Psychiatric Diagnosis is Growing." *Health Affairs* 30(8):1434–42. doi: 10.1377/hlthaff.2010.1024.

National Institute of Mental Health. "The Numbers Count: Mental Disorders in America." www.nimh.nih.gov/health/publications/the-numbers-count-mental-disorders-in-america/index.shtml. Accessed July 26, 2013.

Pratt, Laura A., Debra J. Brody, and Qiuping Gu. 2011. "Antidepressant Use in Persons Aged 12 and Over: United States 2005–2008." *NCHS Data Brief* 76 (October). Atlanta, GA: Center for Disease Control and Prevention. www.cdc.gov/nchs/data/databriefs/db76.htm.

Zajonc, Robert B. 1985. "Emotions and Facial Expression." *Science* 230 (4726): 608–87.

DAY 15

Editors of Publications International. "20 Everyday Activities and the Calories They Burn." *Discovery Fit & Health.* http://health.howstuffworks.com/wellness/diet-fitness/information/20-everyday-activities-and-the-calories-they-burn.htm. Accessed July 26, 2013.

Harvard Medical School. 2004. "Calories Burned in 30 Minutes for People of Three Different Weights." *Harvard Heart Letter* July. www.health.harvard.edu/newsweek/Calories-burned-in-30-minutes-of-leisure-and-routine-activities.htm.

Healy, Genevieve N., David W. Dunstan, Jo Salmon, Ester Cerin, Jonathan E. Shaw, Paul Z. Zimmet, and Neville Owen. 2008. "Breaks in Sedentary Time." *Diabetes Care* 31(4):661–66. doi:10.2337/dc07-2046.

Helmerhorst, Hendrik J. F., Katrien Wijndaele, Soren Brage, Nicholas J. Wareham, and Ulf Ekelund. 2009. "Objectively Measured Sedentary Time May Predict Insulin Resistance Independent of Moderate- and Vigorous-Intensity Physical Activity." *Diabetes* 58(8):1776–79. doi:10.2337/db08-1773.

Levine, James A. 2002. "Non-Exercise Activity Thermogenesis (NEAT)." *Best Practice & Research. Clinical Endocrinology & Metabolism* 16(4):679–702. www.ncbi.nlm.nih.gov/pubmed/12468415.

Levine, James A., Mark W. Vander Weg, James O. Hill, and Robert C. Klesges. 2006. "Non-Exercise Activity Thermogenesis: The Crouching Tiger Hidden Dragon of Societal Weight Gain." *Arteriosclerosis, Thrombosis, and Vascular Biology* 26(4):729–36. doi:10.1161/01.ATV.0000205848.83210.73.

Milanski, Marciane, Ana P. Arruda, Andressa Coope, Leticia M. Ignacio-Souza, Carla E. Nunez, Erika A. Roman, Talita Romanatto, et al. 2012. "Inhibition of Hypothalamic Inflammation Reverses Diet-Induced Insulin Resistance in the Liver." *Diabetes* 61(6):1455–62. doi:10.2337/db11-0390.

Scherer, Thomas, Claudia Lindtner, Elizabeth Zielinski, James O'Hare, Nila Filatova, and Christoph Buettner. 2012. "Short Term Voluntary Overfeeding Disrupts Brain Insulin Control of Adipose Tissue Lipolysis." *Journal of Biological Chemistry* 287 (39): 3061–69. doi:10.1074/jbc.M111.307348.

Shoelson, Steven, Laura Herrero, and Afia Naaz. 2007. "Obesity, Inflammation, and Insulin Resistance." *Gastroenterology* 132:2169–80. doi:10.1053/j.gastro.2007.03.059.

DAY 16

Abu-Taha, May, Cristina Rius, Carlos Hermenegildo, Inmaculada Noguera, Jose-Miguel Cerda-Nicolas, Andrew C. Issekutz, Peter J. Jose, et al. 2009. "Menopause and Ovariectomy Cause a Low Grade of Systemic Inflammation That May be Prevented by Chronic Treatment with Low Doses of Estrogen or Losartan." *Journal of Immunology* 183(2):1393–402. doi:10.4049/jimmunol.0803157.

Chae, Jey Sook, Jean Kyung Paik, Ryungwoo Kang, Minjoo Kim, Yongin Choi, Sang-Hyun Lee, and Jong Ho Lee. 2013. "Mild Weight Loss Reduces Inflammatory Cytokines, Leukocyte Count, and Oxidative Stress in Overweight and Moderately Obese Participants Treated for 3 Years with Dietary Modification." *Nutrition Research* 33(3):195–203. doi: 10.1016/j.nutres.2013.01.005.

Clement, Karine, and Dominique Langin. 2007. "Regulation of Inflammation-Related Genes in Human Adipose Tissue." *Journal of Internal Medicine* 262:422–30. doi: 10.1111/j.1365-2796.2007.01851.x.

Danese, Andrea, Terrie E. Moffitt, Carmine M. Pariante, Antony Ambler, Richie Poulton, and Avshalom Caspi. 2008. "Elevated Inflammation Levels in Depressed Adults with a History of Childhood Maltreatment." *Archives of General Psychiatry* 65:409–16. doi: 10.1001/archpsyc.65.4.409.

Gu, Yei, Shan Yu, and Joshua D. Lambert. 2013. "Dietary Cocoa Ameliorates Obesity-Related Inflammation in High Fat-Fed Mice." *European Journal of Nutrition* published online ahead of print March 15. doi:10.1007/s00394-013-0510-1.

Hooper, Philip L., and Paul L. Hooper. 2009. "Inflammation, Heat Shock Proteins, and Type 2 Diabetes." *Cell Stress & Chaperones* 14(2):113–15. doi:10.1007/s12192-008-0073-x.

Imayama, Ikuyo, Cornelia M. Ulrich, Catherine M. Alfano, Chiachi Wang, Liren Xiao, Mark H. Wener, Kristin L. Campbell, et al. 2012. "Effects of a Caloric Restriction Weight Loss Diet and Exercise on Inflammatory Biomarkers in Overweight/Obese Postmenopausal Women: A Randomized Controlled Trial." *Cancer Research* 72(9): 2314–26. doi:10.1158/0008-5472.CAN-11-3092.

Labonté, Marie-Ève, Patrick Couture, Caroline Richard, Sophie Desroches, and Benoît Lamarche. 2013. "Impact of Dairy Products on Biomarkers of Inflammation: A Systematic Review of Randomized Controlled Nutritional Intervention Studies in Overweight and Obese Adults." *American Journal of Clinical Nutrition* 97(4):706–17. doi:10.3945/ajcn.112.052217.

Lewis, Michael B., and Patrick J. Bowler. 2009. "Botulinum Toxin Cosmetic Therapy Correlates with a More Positive Mood." *Journal of Cosmetic Dermatology* 8(1):24–26. doi:10.1111/j.1473-2165.2009.00419.x.

Massiera, Florence, Pascal Barbry, Philippe Guesnet, Aurélie Joly, Serge Luquet, Chimene Moreilhon-Brest, Tala Mohsen-Kanson, et al. 2010. "A Western-Like Fat Diet Is Sufficient to Induce a Gradual Enhancement in Fat Mass Over Generations." *Journal of Lipid Research* 51(8):2352–61. doi:10.1194/jlr.M006866.

Milanski, Marciane, Ana P. Arruda, Andressa Coope, Leticia M. Ignacio-Souza, Carla E. Nunez, Erika A. Roman, Talita Romanatto, et al. 2012. "Inhibition of Hypothalamic Inflammation Reverses Diet-Induced Insulin Resistance in the Liver." *Diabetes* 61(6):1455–62. doi:10.2337/db11-0390.

Shoelson, Steven, Laura Herrero, and Afia Naaz. 2007. "Obesity, Inflammation, and Insulin Resistance." *Gastroenterology* 132:2169–80. doi:10.1053/j.gastro.2007.03.059.

Thaler, Joshua P., and Michael W. Schwartz. 2010. "Minireview: Inflammation and Obesity Pathogenesis: The Hypothalamus Heats Up." *Endocrinology* 151(9):4109–15. doi:10.1210/en.2010-0336.

DAY 17

Campbell, Peter T., Kristin L. Campbell, Mark H. Wener, Brent L. Wood, John D. Potter, Anne McTiernan, and Cornelia M. Ulrich. 2009. "A Yearlong Exercise

Intervention Decreases CRP among Obese Postmenopausal Women." *Medicine & Science in Sports & Exercise* 41(8):1533–39. doi:10.1249/MSS.0b013e31819c7feb pp.1533-9.

Ford, Earl S. 2002. "Does Exercise Reduce Inflammation? Physical Activity and C-Reactive Protein Among U.S. Adults." *Epidemiology* 13(5):561–68. www.jstor.org/stable/3703940.

Hanh, Thich N. *The Long Road Turns to Joy: A Guide to Walking Meditation* (Berkeley, CA: Parallax Press, 2011), 3.

Ogedegbe, Gbenga O., Carla Boutin-Foster, Martin T. Wells, John P. Allegrante, Alice M. Isen, Jared B. Jobe, and Mary E. Charlson. 2012. "A Randomized Controlled Trial of Positive-Affect Intervention and Medication Adherence in Hypertensive African Americans." *Archives of Internal Medicine* 172(4):322–26. doi:10.1001/archinternmed.2011.1307.

Riesco, Eléonor, Stéphane Choquette, Mélisa Audet, Johann Lebon, Daniel Tessier, and Isabelle J. Dionne. 2012. "Effect of Exercise Training Combined with Phytoestrogens on Adipokines and C-Reactive Protein in Postmenopausal Women: A Randomized Trial." *Metabolism* 61(2):273–80. doi:10.1016/j.metabol.2011.06.025.

Rosenkranz, Melissa A., Richard J. Davidson, Donal G. MacCoon, John F. Sheridan, Ned H. Kalin, Antoine Lutz. 2013. "A Comparison of Mindfulness-Based Stress Reduction and an Active Control in Modulation of Neurogenic Inflammation." *Brain, Behavior, and Immunity* 27(1):174-84. doi:10.1016/j.bbi.2012.10.013.

Suarez, Edward C. 2004. "C-Reactive Protein is Associated with Psychological Risk Factors of Cardiovascular Disease in Apparently Healthy Adults." *Psychosomatic Medicine* 66(5):684–91. doi:10.1097/01.psy.0000138281.73634.67.

Williams, Geoffrey C., and Christopher P. Niemiec. 2012. "Positive Affect and Self-Affirmation Are Beneficial, but Do They Facilitate Maintenance of Health-Behavior Change? Comment on 'A Randomized Controlled Trial of Positive-Affect Intervention and Medication Adherence in Hypertensive African Americans.'" *Archives of Internal Medicine* 172(4):327–28. doi: 10.1001/archinternmed.2011.1830.

Yamamoto, Kazuhiko, Ai Ozazaki, and Susumu Ohmori. 2011. "The Relationship Between Psychosocial Stress, Age, BMI, CRP, Lifestyle, and the Metabolic Syndrome in Apparently Healthy Subjects." *Journal of Physiological Anthropology* 30(1):15-22. http://dx.doi.org/10.211/jpa2.30.15.

Zoccola, Peggy M., Wilson S. Figueroa, Erin M. Rabideau, and Alex Woody. 2013. "Differential Effects of Post-Stressor Rumination and Distraction on C-Reactive Protein in Healthy Women." Paper presented at the 71st Annual Meeting of the American Psychosomatic Society, Miami, FL, March 14–17.

DAY 18

Basaranoglu, Metin, Gokcen Basaranoglu, Tevfik Sabuncu, and Hakan Sentürk. 2013. "Fructose as a Key Player in the Development of Fatty Liver Disease." *World Journal of Gastroenterology* 19(8):1166–72. doi:10.3748/wjg.v19.i8.1166.

Henriksen, Magne, Jørgen Jahnsen, Idar Lygren, Njål Stray, Jostein Sauar, Morten H. Vatn, Bjørn Moum, and the IBSEN Study Group. 2008. "C-Reactive Protein: A Predictive Factor and Marker of Inflammation in Inflammatory Bowel Disease. Results from a Prospective Population-Based Study." *Gut* 57:1518–23. doi:10.1136/gut.2007.146357.

Milanski, Marciane, Ana P. Arruda, Andressa Coope, Leticia M. Ignacio-Souza, Carla E. Nunez, Erika A. Roman, Talita Romanatto, et al. 2012. "Inhibition of Hypothalamic Inflammation Reverses Diet-Induced Insulin Resistance in the Liver." *Diabetes* 61(6):1455–62. doi:10.2337/db11-0390.

DAY 19

Morris, Alanna, Dorothy Coverson, Lucy Fike, Yusuf Ahmed, Neli Stoyanova, W. Craig Hooper, Gary Gibbons, et al. 2010. "Sleep Quality and Duration Are Associated with Higher Levels of Inflammatory Biomarkers: The META-Health Study." Paper presented at the American Heart Association Scientific Sessions, Chicago, November 13–17.

Nedeltcheva, Arlet V., Jennifer M. Kilkus, Jacqueline Imperial, Dale A. Schoeller, and Plamen D. Penev. 2010. "Insufficient Sleep Undermines Dietary Efforts to Reduce Adiposity." *Annals of Internal Medicine* 153(7):435–41. doi:10.7326/0003-4819-153-7-201010050-00006.

Nedeltcheva, Arlet V., Jennifer M. Kilkus, Jacqueline Imperial, Kristin Kasza, Dale A. Schoeller, and Plamen D. Penev. 2009. "Sleep Curtailment Is Accompanied by Increased Intake of Calories from Snacks." *American Journal of Clinical Nutrition* 89(1):126–33. doi:10.3945/ajcn.2008.26574.

St-Onge, Marie-Pierre, Andrew McReynolds, Zalak B. Trivedi, Amy L. Roberts, Melissa Sy, and Joy Hirsch. 2012. "Sleep Restriction Leads to Increased Activation of Brain Regions Sensitive to Food Stimuli." *American Journal of Clinical Nutrition* 95(4):818–24. doi:10.3945/ajcn.111.027383.

Schmid, Sebastian M., Kamila Jauch-Chara, Manfred Hallschmid, and Bernd Schultes. 2009. "Mild Sleep Restriction Acutely Reduces Plasma Glucagon Levels In Healthy Men." *Journal of Clinical Endocrinology and Metabolism* 94(12):5169–73. doi:10.1210/jc.2009-0969.

DAY 20

Chen, Jin Jin, Ren Wang, Xiao-fang Li, and Rui-liang Wang. 2011. "Bifidobacterium Longum Supplementation Improved High-Fat-Fed-Induced Metabolic Syndrome and Promoted Intestinal Reg I Gene Expression." *Experimental Biology and Medicine* 236(7):823–31. doi: 10.1258/ebm.2011.010399.

Kalliomaki, Marko, Maria Carmen Collado, Seppo Salminen, and Erika Isolauri. 2008. "Early Differences in Fecal Microbiota Composition in Children May Predict Overweight." *American Journal of Clinical Nutrition* 87(3):534–38. http://ajcn.nutrition.org/content/87/3/534.long.

Karlsson, Caroline L., Göran Molin, Frida Fak, Marie-Louise Johansson Hagslätt, Maja Jakesevic, Asa Hakansson, Bengt Jeppsson, et al. 2011. "Effects on Weight Gain and Gut Microbiota in Rats Given Bacterial Supplements and a High-Energy-Dense Diet from Fetal Life Through to 6 Months of Age." *British Journal of Nutrition* 106(6):887–95. doi:10.1017/S0007114511001036.

Kondo, Shizuki, Jin-zhong Xiao, Takumi Satoh, Toshitaka Odamaki, Sachiko Takahashi, Kirosuke Sugahara, Tomoko Yaeshima, et al. 2010. "Antiobesity Effects of Bifidobacterium Breve Strain B-3 Supplementation in a Mouse Model with High-Fat Diet-Induced Obesity." *Bioscience, Biotechnology, and Biochemistry* 74(8):1656–61. doi: 10.1271/bbb.100267.

Ley, Ruth E., Fredrik Bäckhed, Peter Turnbaugh, Catherine A. Lozupone, Robin D. Knight, and Jeffrey I. Gordon. 2005. "Obesity Alters Gut Microbial Ecology." *Proceedings of the National Academy of Sciences* 102(31):11070–75. doi: 10.1073/pnas.0504978102.

Mathur, Ruchi, Meridythe Amichai, Kathleen S. Chua, James Mirocha, Gillian M. Barlow, and Mark Pimental. 2013. "Methane and Hydrogen Positivity on Breath Test Is Associated with Greater Body Mass Index and Body Fat." *The Journal of Clinical Endocrinology & Metabolism* 98(4):E698–E702. doi: 10.1210/jc.2012-3144.

Slavin, Joanne. 2013. "Fiber and Prebiotics: Mechanisms and Health Benefits." *Nutrients* 5(4):1417–35. doi:10.3390/nu5041417.

Takemura, Naoki, Takuma Okubo, and Kei Sonoyama. 2010. "Lactobacillus Plantarum Strain No. 14 Reduces Adipocyte Size in Mice Fed High-Fat Diet." *Experimental Biology and Medicine* 235(7):849–56. doi:10.1258/ebm.2010.009377.

Upadhyay, Vaibhav, Valeriy Poroyko, Tae-Jin Kim, Suzanne Devkota, Sherry Fu, Donald Liu, Alexei V. Tumanov, et al. 2012. "Lymphotoxin Regulates Commensal Responses to Enable Diet-Induced Obesity." *Nature Immunology* 13(10):947–53. doi: 10.1038/ni.2403.

Vael, Carl, Stijn L. Verhulst, Vera Nelen, Herman Goossens, and Kristine N. Desager. 2011. "Intestinal Microflora and Body Mass Index During the First Three Years of Life: An Observational Study." *Gut Pathogens* 3(1):8. doi:10.1186/1757-4749-3-8.

Zupancic, Margaret, Brandi L. Cantarel, Zhenqui Liu, Elliott F. Drabek, Kathleen A. Ryan, Shana Cirimotich, Cheron Jones, et al. 2012. "Analysis of the Gut Microbiota in the Old Order Amish and its Relation to the Metabolic Syndrome." *PLoS One* 7(8):e43052. doi:10.1371/journal.pone.0043052.

DAY 21

Schwalfenberg, Gerry K. 2012. "The Alkaline Diet: Is There Evidence That an Alkaline ph Diet Benefits Health?" *Journal of Environmental and Public Health* 2012:727630. doi:10.1155/2012/727630.

DAY 23

Anderson, Richard A. 2003. "Chromium and Insulin Resistance." *Nutrition Research Reviews* 16(2):267–75. http://dx.doi.org/10.1079/NRR200366.

Chaput, Jean-Philippe, Anders Mikael Sjöden, Arne Astrup, Jean-Pierre Després, Claude Bouchard, and Angelo Tremblay. 2010. "Risk Factors for Adult Overweight and Obesity: The Importance of Looking Beyond the 'Big Two.'" *Obesity Facts* 3(5):320–27. doi: 10.1159/000321398.

Joosten, Michel M., Ron T. Gansevoort, Kenneth J. Mukamal, Pim van der Harst, Johanna M. Geleijnse, Edith J.M. Feskens, Gerjan Navis, et al. for the PREVEND Study Group. 2013. "Urinary and Plasma Magnesium and Risk of Ischemic Heart Disease." *The American Journal of Clinical Nutrition* 97(6):1299–1306. doi:10.3945/ajcn.112.054114.

Jorde, Rolf, Monica Sneve, Nina Emaus, Yngve Figenschau, and Guri Grimnes. 2010. "Cross-Sectional and Longitudinal Relation Between Serum 25-Hydroxyvitamin D and Body Mass Index: The Tromsø Study." *European Journal of Nutrition* 49:401–407. doi:10.1007/s00394-010-0098-7.

Larsson, Susanna C. 2013. "Urinary Magnesium Excretion as a Marker of Heart Disease Risk." *The American Journal of Clinical Nutrition* 97 (6):1159–60. doi:10.3945/ ajcn.113.063354.

LeBlanc, Erin S., Joanne H. Rizzo, Kathryn L. Pedula, Kristine E. Ensrud, Jane Cauley, Marc Hochberg, and Teresa A. Hillier, for the Study of Osteoporotic Fractures. 2012. "Associations Between 25-Hydroxyvitamin D and Weight Gain in Elderly Women." *Journal of Women's Health* 21(10):1066–73. doi:10.1089/jwh.2012.3506.

Major, Genevieve C., Francine P. Alarie, Jean Doré, and Angelo Tremblay. 2009. "Calcium Plus Vitamin D Supplementation and Fat Mass Loss in Female Very Low-Calcium Consumers: Potential Link with a Calcium-Specific Appetite Control." *British Journal of Nutrition* 101(5):659–63. doi:10.1017/S0007114508030808.

Maki, Kevin C., Matthew S. Reeves, Mildred Farmer, Koichi Yasunaga, Noboru Matsuo, Yoshihisa Katsuragi, Masanori Komikado, et al. 2009. "Green Tea Catechin Consumption Enhances Exercise-Induced Abdominal Fat Loss in Overweight and Obese Adults." *The Journal of Nutrition* 39(2):264–70. doi: 10.3945/jn.108.098293.

Munro, Irene A., and Manohar L. Garg. 2013. "Prior Supplementation with Long Chain Omega-3 Polyunsaturated Fatty Acids Promotes Weight Loss in Obese Adults: A Double-Blinded Randomised Controlled Trial." *Food & Function* 4(4):650–58. doi:10.1039/c3fo60038f.

Munro, Irene A., and Manohar L. Garg. 2012. "Dietary Supplementation with N-3 PUFA Does not Promote Weight Loss When Combined with a Very-Low-Energy Diet." *British Journal of Nutrition* 108(8):1466–74. doi: 10.1017/S0007114511006817.

Nagao, Tomonori, Tadahi Hase, and Ichiro Tokimitsu. 2007. "A Green Tea Extract High in Catechins Reduces Body Fat and Cardiovascular Risks in Humans." *Obesity* 15(6):1473–83. www.ncbi.nlm.nih.gov/pubmed/17557985.

Okada, Mitsuko, Mayumi Shibuya, Tomoko Akazawa, Hitomi Muya, and Yoko Murakami. 1998. "Dietary Protein as a Factor Affecting Vitamin B6 Requirement." *Journal of Nutritional Science and Vitaminology* 44:37-45. www.ncbi.nlm.nih.gov/pubmed/9591232.

Salas-Salvado, Jordi, Xavier Farrés, Xavier Luque, Silvia Narejos, Manel Borrell, Josep Basora, Anna Anguera, et al. for the Fiber in Obesity-Study Group. 2008. "Effect of Two Doses of a Mixture of Soluble Fibres on Body Weight and Metabolic Variables in Overweight or Obese Patients: A Randomized Trial." *British Journal of Nutrition* 99(6):1380–87. http://dx.doi.org/10.1017/S0007114507868528.

Schirmer, Marie A., and Stephen D. Phinney. 2007. "Gamma-Linolenate Reduces Weight Regain in Formerly Obese Humans." *The Journal of Nutrition* 137(6):1430–35. http://jn.nutrition.org/content/137/6/1430.long.

Shapses, Sue A., Stanley Heshka, and Steven B. Heymsfield. 2004. "Effect of Calcium Supplementation on Weight and Fat Loss in Women." *Journal of Clinical Endocrinology & Metabolism* 89(2):632–37. doi:10.1210/jc.2002-021136.

Sibley, Shalamar D. 2009. "Plasma Vitamin D Predicts Subsequent Weight Loss Success in Overweight Individuals." Paper presented at the 91st Annual Meeting of the Endocrine Society, Washington, DC, June 10–13.

Smeets, Astrid J., Pilou L. H. R. Janssens, and Margriet S. Westerterp-Plantenga. 2013. "Addition of Capsaicin and Exchange of Carbohydrate with Protein Counteract Energy Intake Restriction Effects on Fullness and Energy Expenditure." *The Journal of Nutrition* 143(4):442–47. doi:10.3945/jn.112.170613.

St-Pierre, David H., Rémi Rabasa-Lhoret, Marie-Ève Lavoie, Antony D. Karelis, Irene Strychar, Eric Doucet, and Lise Coderre. 2009. "Fiber Intake Predicts Ghrelin Levels in Overweight and Obese Postmenopausal Women." *European Journal of Endocrinology* 161(1) 65–72. doi:10.1530/EJE-09-0018.

Tremblay, Angelo, and Jo-Anne Gilbert. 2011. "Human Obesity: Is Insufficient Calcium/Dairy Intake Part of the Problem?" *Journal of the American College of Nutrition* 30 (5 Suppl 1):449S–453S. www.jacn.org/content/30/5_Supplement_1/449S.abstract.

Tzotzas, Themistoklis, Fotini G. Papadopoulou, Kostantinos Tziomalos, Spiros Karras, Kostantinos Gastaris, Petros Perros, and Gerasimos E. Krassas. 2010. "Rising Serum 25-Hydroxy-Vitamin D Levels after Weight Loss in Obese Women Correlate with Improvement in Insulin Resistance." *Journal of Clinical Endocrinology and Metabolism* 95(9):4251–57. doi:10.1210/jc.2010-0757.

DAY 24

Holt-Lunstad, Julianne, Timothy B. Smith, and J. Bradley Layton. 2010. "Social Relationships and Mortality Risk: A Meta-Analytic Review." *PLoS Medicine* 7(7): e1000316. doi:10.1371/journal.pmed.1000316.

DAY 25

Atance, Cristina M., and Daniela K. O'Neill. 2005. "The Emergence of Episodic Future Thinking in Humans." *Learning and Motivation* 36:126–44. doi:10.1016/j.lmot.2005.02.003.

Atance, Cristina M., and Daniela K. O'Neill. 2001. "Episodic Future Thinking." *TRENDS in Cognitive Science* 5(12):533–39. www.sciencessociales.uottawa.ca/ccll/fra/documents/15episodicfuturethinking_000.pdf.

Carr, Katelyn A., Tinuke Oluyomi Daniel, Henry Lin, and Leonard H. Epstein. 2011. "Reinforcement Pathology and Obesity." *Current Drug Abuse Reviews* 4(3):190–96. www.ncbi.nlm.nih.gov/pubmed/21999693.

Christakis, Nicholas A., and James H. Fowler. 2007. "The Spread of Obesity in a Large Social Network Over 32 Years." *The New England Journal of Medicine* 357(4):370–79. doi:10.1056/NEJMsa066082.

Hruschka, Daneil J., Alexandra A. Brewis, Amber Wutich, and Benjamin Morin. 2011. "Shared Norms and Their Explanation for the Social Clustering of Obesity." *American Journal of Public Health* 101(Suppl. 1): S295–S300. doi:10.2105/AJPH.2010.300053.

Nielsen 2011 Global Survey. 2012. "Fifty-Nine Percent of Consumers Around the World Indicate Difficulty Understanding Nutritional Labels." www.nielsen.com/us/en/press-room/2012/fifty-nine-percent-of-consumers-around-the-world-indicate-diffic.html. Accessed July 26, 2013.

Peters, Jan, and Christian Büchel. 2010. "Episodic Future Thinking Reduces Reward Delay Discounting Through an Enhancement of Prefrontal-Mediotemporal Interactions." *Neuron* 66(1):138–48. doi:10.1016/j.neuron.2010.03.026.

Shimizu, Mitsuru, Laura E. Smith, and Brian Wansink. 2010. "The Fat Suit Study: When Skinny Companions Lead Us to Eat Healthier." *The FASEB Journal* 24 (Meeting Abstract Suppl): 936.8. www.fasebj.org/cgi/content/meeting_abstract/24/1_MeetingAbstracts/936.8.

DAY 26

Ziglar, Zig. *See You at the Top* (Gretna: Pelican Publishing Company, 1975), 194.

DAY 27

Schlam, Tanya R., Nicole L. Wilson, Yuichi Shoda, Walter Mischel, and Ozlem Ayduk. 2013. "Preschoolers' Delay of Gratification Predicts Their Body Mass 30 Years Later." *The Journal of Pediatrics* 162(1):90–93. doi:10.1016/j.jpeds.2012.06.049.

CHAPTER 9

Feinman, Lawrence, and Charles S. Lieber. 1999. "Ethanol and Lipid Metabolism." *The American Journal of Clinical Nutrition* 70(5):791–92. http://ajcn.nutrition.org/content/70/5/791.full.

Soenen, Stijn, Eveline A. P. Martens, Ananda Hochstenbach-Waelen, Sofie G. T. Lemmens, and Margriet S. Westerterp-Plantenga. 2013. "Normal Protein Intake Is Required for Body Weight Loss and Weight Maintenance, and Elevated Protein Intake for Additional Preservation of Resting Energy Expenditure and Fat Free Mass." *The Journal of Nutrition* 143(5):591–96. doi:10.3945/jn.112.167593.

INDEX

ABOUT THE AUTHORS

Cynthia Stamper Graff is President and CEO of Lindora, one of the largest multisite medical weight-control systems in the United States. A nationally recognized expert in the field of weight management, she has been actively involved in the growth and development of Lindora since 1988. Graff, a leader in integrating technology into the treatment of obesity, has been instrumental in developing Lindora's clinical program as well as the online and by-phone options. For three consecutive years, Lindora has been ranked one of the "Top 500 Women Owned Businesses in America" by *Working Woman* magazine.

Graff is the author of *bodyPRIDE, Lean for Life, Lean for Life Phase One: Weight Loss* and *Lean for Life Phase Two: Lifetime Solutions*. She is also the founder of the Lean for Life Foundation, a nonprofit organization that promotes obesity research and educational programs, and funds weight-control services to selected low-income, morbidly obese men, women and children.

An *Orange County Business Journal* Women In Business as well as Excellence in Entrepreneurship award winner, Graff is a faculty fellow at the Ukleja Center for Ethical Leadership. Graff also received the National Association of Women Business Owners Remarkable Women Lifetime Achievement Award in 2006. She has been a member of the Young Presidents Organization since 1993 and a member of Adaptive Business Leaders since 1998. Graff holds a law degree from York University in Toronto, and a B.S. in business finance from California State University-Long Beach. She resides in Newport Beach, California.

Réginald Allouche, M.D., is a diabetes and weight-loss specialist who also holds postgraduate degrees in biological and medical engineering. Recognized as one of the world's foremost nutrition experts, he is also the founder of KOT, the bestselling brand of gourmet diet foods in Europe. A respected author in France, Dr. Allouche's books include *La Révolution Minceur (The Thinness Revolution,* Michel Lafon, 2003), *Mincir à Satiété (Thinness Through Satiety,* Flammarion, 2009), and *Le Plaisir du Sucre au Risque du Pré-diabète (From Sugar Addiction to Prediabetes Risk,* Editions Odile Jacob, 2013).

As a scientific researcher, he has published major works on diabetes, insulin control and nutrition in hospitals, and is currently concentrating on research in the fields of satiety, fat cell metabolism and gut microflora. His research appears in some of the most prestigious medical journals, including the *American Journal of Clinical Nutrition*.

In the field of diet and nutrition, Dr. Allouche has distinguished himself as one of the world's go-to experts. A frequent guest on French television and radio, Dr. Allouche and/or the KOT products have also been featured in more than 50 mainstream European publications, including the French versions of *Cosmopolitan, ELLE,* and *Marie-Claire.* He is on the Advisory Board of *Santé Magazine,* one of the nation's most popular health and wellness publications with a circulation of nearly 500,000. Internationally renowned, Dr. Allouche was chosen to be the nutritional consultant to the "Club des Chefs des Chefs," a group of chefs to the world's presidents, prime ministers and princes. Originally from Paris, France, Dr. Allouche currently resides in New York. For more information on Dr. Allouche, visit www.drallouche.com.

LEAN FOR LIFE ONLINE PROGRAM

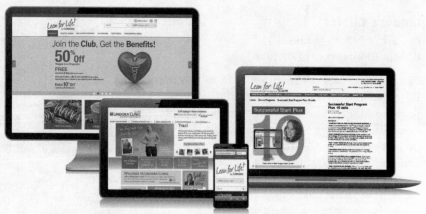

Lean for Life Online provides the day-by-day structure, support and education enjoyed by patients at Lindora's renowned Southern California clinics. When you join this easy-to-use program, you'll enjoy special access to:

- Informative, timely email messages that are specifically relevant to where you are in your program
- Inspiring audio messages
- Charts and graphs that change daily to reflect your progress and keep you motivated
- Forums and chats with Lean for Life program experts
- An extensive online library of Lean for Life videos, recipes... and much more!

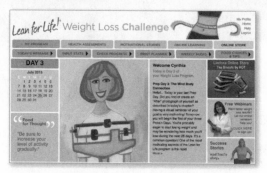

Special Online
Program Offer

Visit www.leanforlife.com or call 1.800.LINDORA to learn more about Lean for Life Online, Lean for Life nutritional products, Lean for Life Coaching by Phone, and Lindora Clinics.

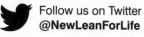 Follow us on Twitter
@NewLeanForLife

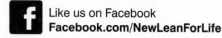 Like us on Facebook
Facebook.com/NewLeanForLife

LEAN FOR LIFE SERVICES

Lindora Clinics

America's Leading Clinical
Weight Management Provider

Founded by Marshall Stamper, M.D. in Newport
Beach, California, Lindora's clinically proven
Lean for Life approach to weight management
has been helping people lose weight and
improve their health since 1971. Lindora's
Lean for Life program, offered at many clinic
locations throughout California, is widely
recognized as the gold standard in medically
supervised weight management.

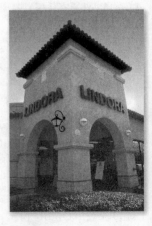

Lean for Life Nutritional Products

- Delicious, nutritious, protein-rich Lean for Life products, specially
  formulated to help satisfy your hunger and control your cravings
- High-quality, cutting-edge vitamins and supplements

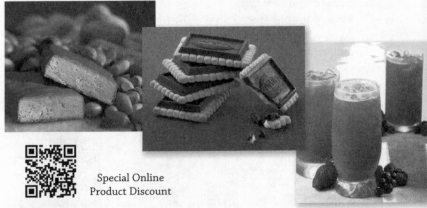

Special Online
Product Discount

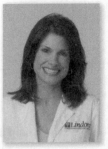

Lean for Life Coaching by Phone

- Get personalized support from Lean for Life experts
- One-on-one, private sessions with friendly,
  experienced coaches
- Guidance, support and motivation for
  maximum results!

lindora.com | 1.800.LINDORA

A MESSAGE TO YOUR DOCTOR

We encourage you to share the following letter with your doctor.

Dear Doctor:

As a physician who has dedicated his career to the treatment of obesity and its co-morbid medical conditions for more than 35 years, I understand how challenging the treatment of obesity can be for both the patient and the physician.

I believe the scientifically sound, common-sense approach of the Lean for Life program offers new hope and a strong, supportive structure to those who want—and need—to lose weight and improve their health. The Lean for Life program is designed to help your patient lose 10% of his or her body weight in ten weeks, and in doing so, significantly reduce their risk for heart disease, diabetes, stroke, hypertension and metabolic syndrome. This book is intended to be both a treatment and therapeutic tool to be used along with your professional guidance.

While *The New Lean for Life* provides your patient with a solid working knowledge of the science of fat loss, you, the physician who best knows the patient, are in a position to be a valuable resource during their weight loss program. For example, there are a number of medications and medication combinations that may be appropriate adjunctive treatment for some patients, but only after your professional assessment can such decisions be made. Lindora has had extensive experience with the use of medications and various therapeutic protocols that have proven to be effective for both weight loss and weight maintenance.

If you would like to receive more information on a medically supervised version of the Lean for Life program, please email us at info@lindora.com.

Best wishes for both you and your patient's success.

Sincerely,

Peter D. Vash, M.D.

Peter D. Vash, M.D., M.P.H.

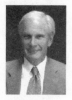

Executive Medical Director, Lindora
Assistant Clinical Professor, UCLA School of Medicine
Past President, American Society of Bariatric Physicians